Amitabh Pandit
Minnie Pandit

super foods
INCREDIBLE IMMUNITY FOR YOUR CHILD

12 WEEKS FOOD PLAN FOR BUILDING A STRONGER IMMUNE SYSTEM

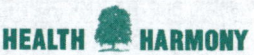

SUPERFOODS – INCREDIBLE IMMUNITY FOR YOUR CHILD

First Edition: 2012
1st Impression: 2012

All rights reserved. No part of this book may be reproduced, stored in a retrieval system or transmitted, in any form or by any means, mechanical, photocopying, recording or otherwise, without any prior written permission of the publisher.

© with the authors

Published by Kuldeep Jain for

HEALTH HARMONY

An imprint of
B. JAIN PUBLISHERS (P) LTD.
An ISO 9001: 2000 Certified Company
1921/10, Chuna Mandi, Paharganj, New Delhi 110 055 (INDIA)
Tel.: +91-11-4567 1000 • Fax: +91-11-4567 1010
Email: info@bjain.com • Website: www.bjain.com

Printed in India by
J.J. Offset Printers

ISBN: 978-81-319-1163-1

CONTENTS

Publisher's Note — v
Disclaimer — ix
Acknowledgements — xi
A Word about Gender — xiii
For Your Shopping Basket — xv

PART I
THE CURTAIN RISES

1. Top 5 Reasons for Missing School — 3
2. Mom's Beware — 12
3. From 'Yuck' to 'Wow' — 25
4. Enter the Food Warriors — 37
5. 3 Pandit Principles — 46
6. Play or Perish — 48
7. 7 Signs of Perfect Health — 54

PART II
THE 12 WEEKS INCREDIBLE IMMUNITY PLAN

1. Week One — 61
2. Week Two — 62
3. Week Three — 63

PART III
FOOD FOR LIFE

Nature's Bounty–Fruits	67
Fascinating World of Spices	80
Tools of Health–Vegetables	87
Your Pot-Pourri	102
Tools For Immunity Building	119
1. Liquid Gold	120
2. Fruit Mélanges	127
3. Plate of Panacea	134
4. The Salad Pot	145
5. Evening Rechargers	160
6. Magic Meals	167
7. Mixed Bag	195
8. Magnify Your Gains	202
Glossary	213
References	219

PUBLISHER'S NOTE

The Winner of 2 International awards and the authors of *Super Foods: Make Your Child a Genius* by B Jain Publishers, Amitabh Pandit and Minnie Pandit, have authored this book for us. They are people who preach what they teach. They are the pioneers of orthomolecular science on the eastern side of the globe, bringing the latest, cutting edge information in the field of anti-ageing, wellness and superior fitness. They say that ignorance regarding–body chemistry, nutrition and a healthy lifestyle leads to poor nutritional choices, chemical deficiencies and diseases like cancer, heart diseases and diabetes. The diseases have taken a terrible toil on life in the developed countries. The authors say that the right kind of knowledge can always lead to a better life, no matter what physical or mental handicaps we have.

Orthomolecular nutrition is a radical science which changes the way people eat and feed their children. This has given wondrous results to people who have taken to it. Many fruits, nuts, seeds, vegetables and diary products can be used to bring about a dramatic change in the body within a short span of time.

This book can assist you as a guidepost to help you feed your children better and pass through some of those periods when you do not know what to give them. Develop your children so as to make them reach their fullest potential.

Kuldeep Jain
C.E.O., B. Jain Publishers (P) Ltd.

OTHER TITLES BY AMITABH PANDIT AND MINNIE:
ANTI-AGEING EXOTIC BLENDS
SUPERFOODS – MAKE YOUR CHILD A GENIUS

Dedication

For the love of children . . .

DISCLAIMER

Information contained in this book is intended as an educational aid only. Information is not intended as medical advice for individual conditions or treatment and is not a substitute for a medical examination, nor does it replace the need for services provided by medical professionals or independent determinations. A person's individual doctor must determine what is safe and effective for each individual person or patient.

While the authors have tested and obtained remarkable results with the foods described herein, the health of a person's digestive system along with his age is a determinant of how well even the best of food is digested and the benefits got from it. Whatever be the case it is important to understand what nutrients can do and from which foods the same can be obtained.

ACKNOWLEDGEMENTS

Our ultimate appreciation must go to the pioneering scientists who use their talents, imagination and energy to study the age-old secrets of food's medicinal powers and how to apply them to today's critical health problems. Our work is a distillation of their many years of work, creativity and discovery.

A WORD ABOUT GENDER

The chances are just about equal that your child is a boy or a girl. Unfortunately, English language does not have a singular pronoun that includes both genders. We did not wish to refer to children as 'it' and we find 'he/she' too awkward. To give equal importance to both sexes, we have, therefore, used the feminine 'she' and 'her' and the masculine 'he', 'him', and 'his' interchangeably in all the chapters.

FOR YOUR SHOPPING BASKET

We have given you a comprehensive list of all the ingredients used in this book. Start by stocking your pantry with these and you will be able to make all the recipes given in the FOOD FOR LIFE section.

VEGETABLES

ENGLISH	HINDI
Baby Corn	Baby Makai
Beetroot	Chukandar
Bottle Gourd	Lauki ya Doodhi
Carrots	Gajar
Cauliflower	Phool Gobhi
Celery	Celery ke Patte
Cherry Tomato	Cherry Tamatar
Corn on the Cob	Sabut Makai ya Bhuttaa
Cucumber	Kheera
French Beans	France Beans ya Hari Beans
Garlic	Lehsun
Ginger Root	Adrak ki Ganth
Green Bell Pepper	Hari Shimla Mirch
Green Cabbage	Hari Patta Bandha Gobhi
Green Chilli	Hari Mirch
Green Lettuce	Hara Salad Patta
Green Peas	Hare Matar
Green Pumpkin	Hara Kaddu
Iceberg Lettuce	Iceberg Salad Patta
Indian Gooseberry	Amla
Karaunda	Karaunda
Lemon	Nimboo
Lotus Root	Kamal Kakri ya Jad
Potato	Aalloo
Radish	Safed Mooli
Raw Papaya	Kachcha Papita
Red Beans	Lal France Beans
Red Bell Pepper	Lal Shimla Mirch (Meethi)
Red Cabbage	Red Patta Bandha Gobhi
Red Lettuce	Lal Salad Patta
Red Radish	Lal Mooli
Spinach	Palak ke Patte
Spring Onion	Hari Pyaaz
Sweet Corn	Meethi Makai
Tomato	Tamatar
Turnip	Shalgam
Yellow Bell-pepper	Peeli Shimla Mirch (Meethi)
Zucchini	Ek kism ki tori

FRUITS

ENGLISH	HINDI
Apples	Seb
Bananas	Kela
Dates	Khajoor
Dry Apricots	Sookhi Khurmani
Figs	Sookhi Anjeer
Kiwi	Kiwi Phal
Mangoes	Aam
Melon	Kharbooja
Munakka	Munakka
Orange	Santra
Papaya	Papita
Pear	Nashpati
Pineapple	Ananas

Pomegranate	Anar
Stone Fruit	Bael phal
Strawberries	Strawberries

GRAINS AND PULSES

ENGLISH	HINDI
Barley Flour	Jau ka atta
Brown Chick Peas	Kala Chana
Brown Rice/ Unpolished Rice	Bhura Chawal
Dry Green Peas	Sookha Hara Matar
Gram Flour	Besan
Green Mung Beans	Sabut Mung Dal
Moth Beans	Sabut Moth Dal
Multigrain Bread	Do Anaaj ki Bread
Red Lentils	Lal Masoor Dal
Semolina	Sooji
Soya Flour	Soya Bean ka Atta
Soybeans	Soya Bean
Vermicelli	Sevain
White Oats	Safed Jai
White Peas	Sookhi Safed Matar
Whole Wheat Bread	Gehun ke Atte ki Bread
Whole Wheat Flour	Gehun ka Atta

SPICES, HERBS AND SEEDS

ENGLISH	HINDI
Aniseeds	Saunf ke beej
Asafoetida	Heeng
Basil Leaves	Tulsi ke Patte
Bay Leaf	Tej Patta
Bishops Weed Seeds	Ajwain ke Beej
Black Mustard Seeds/Powder	Kali Sarson ke Beej/Powder Pisi Kali Sarson
Black Pepper Corns	Kali Mirch ke Dane
Black Salt	Kala Namak
Brown Cardamom	Badi Elaichi
Caraway Seeds	Shahi Jeera
Cardamom	Hari Elaichi
Cinnamon	Dalchini
Cloves	Laung
Coriander Leaves	Dhania Patti
Coriander Seeds/Powder	Dhania ke Beej ya Powder
Cumin Seeds/Powder	Jeera ke Beej ya Powder
Curry Leaves	Kadi Patta Meethi Neem
Curry Powder	Curry Powder
Dry Ginger Powder	Saunth Powder
Garam Masala	Garam Masala
Dried Fenugreek Leaves	Kasoori Methi
Lemon Grass	Zarakhush Ghaas
Melon Seeds	Kharbooje ke Beej
Mint Leaves	Pudina Patti
Nutmeg Powder	Jaiphal ka Powder
Oregano	Ajwain ke Patte
Parsley	Ajmod
Poppy Seeds	Khus Khus
Red Chili Powder	Lal Mirch Powder
Rosemary Leaves	Rosemary ke Patte
Salt	Namak
Sāmbhar Powder	Sambar Powder
Sesame Seeds	Til ke Beej
Sunflower Seeds	Surajmukhi ke Beej

Tamarind	Imli
Thai Ginger	Thailand ki Adrak
Thyme	Thyme ke Patte
Turmeric	Haldi
Vanilla Bean/Extract	Vanilla ka Bean ya Arak
White Pepper	Safed Mirch
Yellow Mustard Seeds	Peeli Sarson ke Beej

Note on herbs usage: You have an advantage with using herbs in this book. They are available throughout the year in fresh or dried form. Anytime a recipe calls for using a herb, use the type you have on hand. Dried herbs are now commonly available at good grocery stores.

Curry powder: Curry powder is a seasoning blend often made with up to 20 different ground spices. It almost always contains turmeric, which is what gives curry powder its' distinct yellow colour. Ranging from mild to very spicy, heat levels vary by brand.

Sambar powder: A mixture of spices specially made for seasoning south Indian cuisine. It includes coriander seeds, asafoetida, red chilies, curry leaves, channa dhal, urad dhal, whole black peppers, fenugreek seeds.

Garam masala: This easy-to-make spice blend is the heart of most Indian dishes. A combination of different spices, it probably has as many recipes as there are families in India! A basic one will include coriander seeds, cumin seeds, black peppercorns, **black cumin seeds, dry ginger**, black cardamom, cloves, cinnamon and **bay leaves**.

ASSORTMENT

ENGLISH	HINDI
Almonds	Badam
Baking Powder	Baking soda
Bread Crumbs	Bread ka Choora
Chicken	Murga
Coconut	Nariyal
Curd/Yoghurt	Dahi
Egg	Anda
Eno Salt	Eno Namak
Extra Virgin Olive Oil	Kachi Dhani se Jaitun ka Tel
Green Olives	Hara Jaitun Phal
Honey	Shehad
Hung Curd	Paani Nikala Hua - Dahi
Olive Oil	Jaitun ka Tel
Peanuts	Mungphali
Prawns/Shrimps	Jhinga
Sesame Oil	Til ka Tel
Soy Sauce	Soya Sauce
Sugar	Cheeni
Tahini	Safed Til ki Chutney/Paste
Tofu	Soya Bean ka Paneer
Water	Paani
Yeast	Khameera

part 1
THE CURTAIN RISES

'Whatever was the father of a disease, an ill-diet was the mother.' – Chinese Proverb

The old saying **'what you don't know can't hurt you' just isn't true** when it comes to body chemistry, nutrition, and a healthy lifestyle. Ignorance leads to poor nutritional choices, chemical deficiencies, and the kinds of diseases that prey on an undernourished and malnourished body and shorten the life span. Heart disease, cancer, and diabetes all have taken a terrible toll on life in the developed countries, and all three of them are strongly influenced by food patterns and lifestyle habits. The right kind of knowledge can always lead us to a better life, no matter what physical or mental handicaps we have.

If you have been following stereotyped food patterns passed down through your family for generations, or have been following cultural traditions about what and how your children should eat, it is never too late to study body chemistry and follow a higher pathway to better health.

Generally, the way to raise healthy children is to follow your intuition and use common sense. The best barometer of your infant's or child's wellbeing is your observation of his growth, physically, mentally, and spiritually. Does he react quickly to different stimuli? Does it seem that she is growing and developing with a natural inquisitiveness and an explorer's heart? Watch for infants who are overly quiet (Oh! How well behaved he is!), or extremely aggressive. And, of course, do not be afraid to seek opinions regarding the health of your children from others, within and without the nutritional community. In your search for information, it can be useful to follow the advice of many health care practitioners: Take charge, be on top of things, be voracious in your appetite for knowledge, and do not ever give away your freedom to choose. In short, take responsibility for your children's lives until they are able to take responsibility themselves.

Orthomolecular nutrition, a radical science changing the way people eat and feed their children has been giving wondrous results to all who have taken to it. It transforms a child's body and makes him look as shapely as a teen idol with glowing skin, lustrous hair, strong immunity, increased efficiency, and brain function, balanced hormonal system with reduced fatigue and without disease.

Many specific fruits, nuts, seeds, vegetables and dairy products can be used to bring about this dramatic change in the young body within a short span of time. These have been put in a coordinated way to formulate **'the 12 weeks incredible immunity plan'.** This simple yet scientific 12 weeks plan can prove to be one of the best and most effective things your child can do this year and year after and year after.

SAME FOOD-SPECIFIC MIXES

'The immunity plan' promotes eating tasty foods, without any quantity restrictions, including delicious fruit mélanges, delectable sherbets, luscious hot and cold drinks, fusion salads and many more lip smacking tiffin's, besides the magic meals to serve on weekends – all quick to make and nutritious. The key behind the final result obtained from the plan is foods consumed in the CORRECT COMBINATIONS. Magical results can be achieved within weeks, while enjoying the enchanting aromas, flavours, textures, and tastes. Your updated knowledge on the breakthroughs in orthomolecular nutrition may change the way you look at human nutrition and get smart to plan food for mealtimes.

This book can assist you as a guidepost to help you feed your children better and pass through some of those periods when you don't know what to give them (they turn up their nose to most foods!). Please enjoy these pages and most of all, pursue your role as a parent so that the development of your children can reach it's fullest potential.

1 TOP 5 REASONS FOR MISSING SCHOOL

Children are precious; as parents you worry about their health. When our children have issues and crises, these issues and crises affect us just as much, if not more, than it affects them. We fear that which might bring them fear; we hurt when we see them hurt; and sometimes, we cry just seeing them cry. It is aptly said, "Making the decision to have a child is momentous. It is to decide forever to have your heart go walking around outside your body." So, when it seems like something is not quite right with your children – perhaps they seem to fall sick more frequently than other kids, they seem to miss school more than their playmates or just don't have enough strength for any activity after attending school - this weak or falling sick syndrome can be experienced as terrifying. In fact, a child's difficulty can be just the starting point for your parental worry and concern. You might not know what to do to help your child, or where to go for help. Possibly, you may worry because you don't even know if your child's problem is something you should be concerned about in the first place.

Today more and more parents are realizing that the key to a healthy child is a strong immune system. All children are constantly exposed to disease producing organisms such as bacteria, viruses, fungi, and parasites but this doesn't mean they will get sick. A strong immune system provides a child with the natural defenses to fight off disease.

If a child has a weakened immune system, he is more susceptible to colds, flu, and other problems. Germs are everywhere and being exposed to them is a natural part of life. It is not natural, however, to try and 'germ proof' your child. Exposure to different viruses and bacteria can actually strengthen your child's immune system. The immune system begins developing before a child is born. A combination of innate resistance to certain diseases, maternally acquired antibodies and active exposure to germs helps build children's immune systems as they grow into adults.

UNDERSTANDING YOUR CHILD'S IMMUNE SYSTEM

Immune systems vary from person to person; some are stronger and some weaker. The immune system protects the body from disease and infection. It attacks dangerous germs that enter the body and fights them off. This is called the immune response. There are three different types of immune responses: Innate, adaptive and passive.

1. We're born with innate, or natural immunity to certain diseases; for example, we can't catch certain ailments animals suffer from. Our skin and mucous membranes, like the inside of our noses, mouths, and intestines, also make up our natural immune system – they are barriers guarding the body against infection.

2. Active, or adaptive immunity develops as you age. The older you get, the more germs you become immune to because you've been exposed to more of them.

3. Passive immunity is borrowed from a different source. A child receives antibodies through his mother's milk, for example. Passive immunity doesn't last very long. You can receive what's called 'passive' inoculation if you're already infected with a particular disease or if you've been exposed to it. This type of inoculation will help you fight off the disease you already have, rather than prevent you from getting it in the first place. It's usually done with serum containing antibodies from immune people (often gamma globulin) or animals.

The immune system begins to develop from stem cells when an embryo is about 5 weeks old. When a baby is born, his immune system is stimulated by the new germs he's exposed to, and he begins to produce antibodies roughly 6 days after birth. He's already temporarily immune to some diseases, because his mother has given him passive immunity while he was in utero. If he's nursing, he'll also be receiving antibodies through her milk. This type of passive immunity, called maternal immunity, will slowly fade over about 6-8 months.

His own immune system will keep growing, and by the time he's 1 year old, he'll already have adult-level immunity to some diseases. He'll still constantly be exposed to new germs, however; if a cold is going around, an adult's body might already have 'learned' how to fight it off, while the same cold might have a baby sniffling and sneezing because he's encountering the germ for the first time.

HEALTH ISSUES IN CHILDHOOD OFTEN SHOW UP IN ADULTHOOD

Physical and mental health problems in childhood can have lifelong consequences, which mean it's important to start health promotion and disease prevention early in life. "A scientific consensus is emerging that the origins of adult disease are often found among developmental and biological disruptions occurring during the early years of life," according to Dr Jack P. Shonkoff, of Harvard University.

Investigators have postulated that early experience can affect adult health in at least two ways – by accumulating damage over time or by the biological embedding of adversities during sensitive developmental periods. In both cases, there can be a lag of many years, even decades, before early adverse experiences are expressed in the form of illness. In a cumulative process, chronic diseases occur as the result of repeated physical and mental stress.

Strong associations have been shown between retrospective adult reports of increasing numbers of traumatic childhood events with greater prevalence of a wide array of health impairments including coronary artery disease, chronic pulmonary disease, cancer, alcoholism, depression, and drug abuse, as well as overlapping mental health problems, teen pregnancies, and cardiovascular risk factors such as obesity, physical inactivity, and smoking.

These findings show that biological embedding of risk factors for poor health can occur during sensitive periods when a child's developing brain is more receptive to a variety of input, both positive and negative.

THE TOP FIVE CULPRITS

There are many days of your child's young life that he will be missing school due to illness. Do you know why children get sick so often? Or when it's safe to send kids back to school or child care? In school or child care, your child's immune system is put to the test. After all, young children in large groups are breeding grounds for the organisms that cause illness.

COMMON COLD

Most people catch several colds each year, usually in the fall, winter, and spring. Common cold spreads easily through contact with infected respiratory droplets coughed or sneezed into the air. When your child catches a cold, after he has been exposed to cold viruses being spread by some other person, you may sneeze, feel a chill and scratchiness of the throat, develop a runny nose or a stopped up nose, or may feel rather miserable for two or three days.

Signs and symptoms may include swollen tonsils, cough, sneezing, and low grade fever, or high fever depending upon severity. At this time it is usually wise to stay at home and rest in bed, for his own wellbeing and to spare his family and colleagues the risk of exposure to his cold. It usually takes 7-10 days before he will fully recover.

Having a cold 2-3 times a year is not pleasant. What is worse, the cold may be attended by serious complications – bronchitis, sinus infection, infection of the middle ear, infection of the mastoid bone (mastoiditis), meningitis, bronchopneumonia, or lobar pneumonia.

In medical literature, nonetheless, it continues to be said that no clearly effective method of treatment of common cold has been developed. The various drugs that are prescribed or recommended have some value in making the patient more comfortable, by giving relief from some of the more distressing symptoms, but they have little effect on the duration of the cold. The fact that doctors have not had a good way of preventing and treating common cold has been the subject of many jokes.

Nutrition quotient: Incorrect dietary habits are often the root cause of frequent colds in children. The prevalent excessive use of dairy products including milk, curd, cheese, and ghee can clog the tender respiratory systems of kids. Current research shows that these foods can lead to formation of thickened mucous, especially in lactose intolerant children. If your child does not show symptoms of lactose intolerance and still bears a perpetual cold, runny nose or cough, it will be a sound decision to avoid these foods for a month and observe for improvements.

VIRAL GASTROENTERITIS

This is an inflammation of the stomach and intestines from a virus and sometimes called the 'stomach flu'. These viruses are often found in contaminated food and drinking water, or typically develop after contact with an infected person. Symptoms of viral gastroenteritis usually appear within 4 - 48 hours of exposure to the contaminated food or water. The signs to watch out for are abdominal pain, diarrhoea, nausea, vomiting. There might also be chills, clammy skin, excessive sweating, and fever.

Parents must look for dry or sticky mouth, excessive lethargy, low or no urine output and markedly sunken soft spots (fontanelles) on the top of an infant's head. Antibiotics do not work for viruses, hence there's no effective medical treatment for viral gastroenteritis. Drugs to slow down the amount of diarrhoea (anti-diarrhoeal medications) should not be given without first talking with your paediatrician. These medications can make it harder for your child's body to eliminate the virus and may cause the infection to last longer.

Nutrition quotient: The goal of treatment is to prevent dehydration by making sure the body has as much water and fluids as it should. Fluids and electrolytes (salt and minerals) lost through diarrhoea or vomiting must be replaced by drinking extra fluids. Avoid using fruit juices, fresh or packed since all of these have a lot of sugar, which makes diarrhoea worse, and they don't replace lost minerals. Get your child to drink small amounts of fluid every 30-60 minutes, rather than trying to force large amounts at one time, which can cause vomiting. Use a teaspoon or syringe for an infant or a small child. Encourage your child to rest as much as possible and never force feed at this stage. The idea of keeping up strength by eating heartily backfires in gastroenteritis and weakens the system further. Giving easy-to-digest items such as soups, toast, and vegetables can lead to faster recovery. Gradually, you can return to the normal diet of cereals, legumes, dairy, and meat.

EAR INFECTION (OTITIS MEDIA)

Ear infections usually start with a viral infection, such as a cold. The middle ear becomes inflamed from the infection, and fluid builds up behind the eardrum. This fluid can become a breeding ground for viruses or bacteria. A parent should suspect ear infection when the child complains of ear pain, tugs, or pulls at the affected ear, be unusually irritable or have trouble sleeping. Ear infections can be a disabling disease for young ones since it might be accompanied by a fever also.

Until recently, all children with ear infections were given antibiotics. New research suggests that many children with ear infections will get better without antibiotics, and with no ill-effects. This is called the 'observation option'. This option reduces the use of unnecessary antibiotics, and limits the child's exposure to the side effects of antibiotics. It also reduces the chance that 'super bacteria' — bacteria that cannot be killed by antibiotics — will develop. If your child is uncomfortable, you can ask your child's doctor about pain relievers. He or she may recommend eardrops or an over-the-counter pain reliever.

Ear infections are not contagious nor can they spread from one person to another, but the colds that result in ear infections are. Colds are spread when germs are released from the nose or mouth during coughing or sneezing. Anything that can reduce the spread of germs will help reduce ear infections.

Nutrition quotient: Cold foods like ice creams and colas can increase the symptoms of an ear infection. Sugary foods like breakfast cereals, chocolates, cakes and pastries weaken the digestive system and lower immunity. Frequent consumption of such foods can result in viral infections and influenza, the precursor to ear infections. No one should be allowed to smoke around children. Secondhand smoke increases a child's risk for ear infections.

ALLERGIES

An allergy is an over-reaction of the immune system to a substance that's harmless to most people. But in someone with an allergy, the body's immune system treats the substance (called an allergen) as an invader and reacts inappropriately, resulting in symptoms that can be anywhere from annoying to possibly harmful to the person.

In a child with allergies, the first exposure to an allergen stimulates the immune system to recognize the substance. Any exposure after that will usually result in symptoms. When an allergen enters the body of a person who has sensitized the immune system, certain cells release histamine and other chemicals. This causes itching, swelling, mucous production, muscle spasms, hives, rashes, and other symptoms.

The body part that comes in direct contact with the allergen will affect symptoms. For example, inhaled allergens will cause nasal congestion, itchy nose and throat, mucous production, coughing, or wheezing. In general, food allergies may cause abdominal pain, cramping, diarrhoea, nausea, or vomiting. Frequently plant allergies cause skin rash and drug allergies involve the whole body. Some of the chronic diseases related to allergies are eczema and asthma. Common allergens for children include dust mites, pollen, moulds, pets, cockroaches, peanuts, cow's milk, soy, insect stings, antibiotics, and chemicals in cosmetics, or detergents.

Conventional medical science offers no real cure for allergies, but can assist in relieving symptoms. Medications prescribed include antihistamines and steroids depending upon the type of allergy. The only real way according to the old school is to cope with allergies by reducing or eliminating exposure to allergens.

Nutrition quotient: Eat away your allergies. British scientists surveyed the parents of nearly 700 children in the Greek island of Crete to assess their respiratory symptoms and dietary habits. They found that at least twice a day, eight out of 10 children ate fresh fruit, and two-thirds ate fresh vegetables. The health benefits appeared to be strongest in terms of respiratory problems. Children who followed this healthy diet were less likely to develop air or skin allergies, or asthma symptoms. According to the scientists, these foods provide the maximum benefits based on their antioxidant properties. Antioxidants are known for their disease-fighting ability. They work to sop-up the free radicals left over in the body as a byproduct of a cell's day-to-day functions.

They concluded that eating a nutritional diet, one that is rich in vegetables, fruits, and whole grains, will help protect against allergies and asthma.

IRRITABLE BOWEL SYNDROME

IBS or irritable bowel syndrome is among the most troublesome diseases in daily life. Also referred to by the concept of functional bowel disorder it does not spare children. "Mom, I have a stomachache", is one of the biggest complaints heard by parents.

To have a bowel movement, the muscles in the colon and the rest of the body have to work together. If this process is somehow interrupted, the contents of the colon can't move along very smoothly. It sort of stops and starts, doesn't move, or sometimes moves too fast. This can hurt and make a child feel awful. Children with IBS may have more sensitive bowels, so what might cause a little discomfort in one person causes serious pain for someone with IBS. Between 5 per cent to 20 per cent of children have IBS but the good news is that it doesn't lead to more serious problems.

The symptoms to look for will be occasional stomachache along with constipation (hard stools that make it difficult to go to the bathroom) or diarrhoea (stools that are really loose and watery). A child with IBS may sometimes feel like he or she can't quite finish going to the bathroom. Or, if he or she has gas, instead of passing it, it may feel trapped inside.

According to the traditional medical school of thought, no one really knows what causes IBS. The only cause understood till now seems to be stress. Stress can speed up your colon and slow your stomach down. In severe cases, the doctor might give a person some medicine for IBS to reduce pain, as well as help manage gas, constipation, diarrhoea, and the need to rush to the bathroom.

There is no test to diagnose IBS. Doctors often diagnose the problem just by listening to a person describe the symptoms. That's why it's really important for kids to talk with their parents and their doctor about their symptoms — even if it seems embarrassing.

Nutrition quotient: Parents need not panic on account of IBS. This condition is transitory and these problems diminish or disappear as they grow. Still it is one of the leading reasons for visits to the doctor's clinic and should be attended to relieve the child. Several other causes are now attributed to the cause of this menace – antibiotics, excessive weakness, lack of exercise but 3 out of 4 cases of IBS can be related to errors in diet.

Most often, this is a diet high in refined carbohydrates like sugar, white flour, and excess protein (meat, fish, eggs). Beware, it's not just what a child eats — what he or she doesn't eat also may lead to IBS symptoms. Fruits, vegetables, and high fibre foods like whole grains and beans can help keep a child's colon running properly.

RESISTANCE TO ANTIBIOTICS IS BECOMING A BIG PROBLEM

Antibiotics, first used in the 1940s may be one of the great advances in medicine. But overprescribing them has resulted in the development of bacteria that doesn't respond to antibiotics that may have worked in the past. Besides, children who take antibiotics when they aren't necessary run the risk of adverse reactions, such as stomach upset and diarrhoea.

You can play the role of a responsible parent by understanding how antibiotics work. There are two major types of germs that can make people sick: Bacteria and viruses. Although certain bacteria and viruses cause diseases with similar symptoms, the ways these two organisms multiply and spread illness are different:

Bacteria are *living* organisms existing as single cells. These are everywhere and most don't cause any harm, and in some cases may be beneficial. Lactobacillus, for example, lives in the intestine and helps digest food. But some bacteria are harmful and can cause illness by invading the human body, multiplying, and interfering with normal bodily processes. Antibiotics are effective against bacteria because they work to kill these living organisms by stopping their growth and reproduction.

Viruses, on the other hand, are not alive and cannot exist on their own. They are particles containing genetic material wrapped in a protein coat. Viruses 'live', grow, and reproduce only after they've invaded other living cells. Some viruses may be fought off by the body's immune system before they cause illness, but others (colds, for example) must simply run their course. Viruses do not respond to antibiotics at all.

Taking antibiotics for colds and other viral illnesses not only won't work, but also has a dangerous side effect. Over a time period, this practice helps create bacteria that have become more of a challenge to kill. Frequent and inappropriate use of antibiotics breeds strains of bacteria that can resist treatment. This is called bacterial resistance. These resistant bacteria require higher doses of medicine or stronger antibiotics to treat. Doctors have even found bacteria that are resistant to some of the most powerful antibiotics available today.

Antibiotic resistance is a widespread problem, and one that the U.S. Centres for Disease Control and Prevention calls "one of the world's most pressing public health problems." Each time you give antibiotics to your children, you increase the likelihood of their getting a disease caused by resistant bacteria.

NEW DANGERS OF MEDICATION

Every drug you use will leave residues of some kind in your child's body even after he quits taking it. While you are using prescription and over-the-counter remedies, these drugs mix with the chemical food additives he consumes when he eats processed foods, together with bile salts, pancreatic enzymes, putrefying proteins, the metabolic by-products, and bowel bacteria. The bowel, lymph, blood stream, and liver can become a kind of catchall system, not necessarily able to detoxify or excrete all the chemically harmful substances that interact with one another as well as with the body chemistry. Often, toxic substances are stored in body fat, genetically weak organs, amid tissues, and the bones.

Tissue cleansing to get rid of all this repugnant debris is one of the best approaches to developing a healthier body. I put children coming to me on a diet that is half cleansing (getting rid of stored toxins) and half building (repairing damaged tissue). What they have done with their body in the past will determine how hard they will have to work to cleanse and rebuild their body.

Drugs are simpler and more convenient to administer, but they all initiate unnatural reactions or harmful biological reactions (especially steroids and antibiotics) in the body. We are not opposed to using drugs to save lives when there is no effective alternative therapy, but everyone who uses drugs – prescription, over-the-counter, or street drugs – is introducing chemicals into his or her body that the body was never designed to assimilate or process. Often, the liver enzymes have to break down or detoxify, at least part of most drugs.

I favour a natural and gentler approach to health whenever possible because so many of the prescriptions and therapies of our time leave children at a lower level of health than before treatment. Foods don't do that. I believe that the balancing of body chemistry by selected nutrients will become the obvious and preferable means of restoring the functioning of enzyme reaction sequences, thus bringing about restored function at the level of organs, glands, and tissues.

DISEASE FIGHTING POWER OF FOOD

However common they may be, childhood disorders are not part of the normal developmental process that children are expected to go through. Today scientists with new technology can detect, isolate, and test minute quantities of bioactive plant compounds. Using sophisticated laboratory tests, they are ferreting out the biological activities of whole foods, their constituents, and their impact on disease processes.

Scientists are also scrutinizing the diets of populations with low rates of disease – for example, Mediterranean people and the Japanese to determine how they eat differently from people with high disease rates. In 'case-control' studies, nearly identical groups of individuals are studied, except one group has a particular disease and the other does not, then their diets are compared. A lot of clues come from such so-called epidemiological or population studies.

The best are intervention studies, in which researchers actually put people with a certain malady, such as heart disease or precancerous lumps, on very specific but different diets. They then keep track of who gets worse or better in the next 2-3 years. In this way a food is tested much like a drug to judge the potency of the therapy. Such intervention studies are rare, but the advice derived from them is golden. The same golden advice has been used to produce recipes in Part III of this book 'Food for life'. Using this knowledge as your child gets older, he will build an arsenal of antibodies to fight common diseases, will become less prone to childhood illnesses and recover more quickly from the ones he does catch.

2 MOM'S BEWARE

The recognition of deficiency diseases was a major breakthrough that established nutrition as a medical science. Even though modern medical education has now started appreciating nutrition considering it just as crucial as anatomy, physiology, biochemistry, and pharmacology to understanding human health, much still needs to be done to make it a part of the curriculum.

In the current state of knowledge, highlight has fallen on the role of certain foods either as risk factors or as protectors against disease. Diets and dietetics recommend 'good food eating practices' for everyone and specific measures for the sick or those who want to lose a few pounds. But nutrition is a huge scientific field to explore and research is in full swing throughout the world on complex topics such as the nutritional needs of the organization, the role of genetic factors on nutritional status and the mode of action of nutrients and their specific effect on the onset of disease. Therefore in the years to come recommendations on nutrition will get even more importance and become more accurate in terms of prevention and treatment of diseases.

What roles does a given nutrient play in the body? How much of it do we need? What is the optimum amount of this nutrient? (Every constituent of our body – sodium, iron, glucose – has an optimum level.) The answers would probably reveal that most of us fall at the low end of the nutrient intake curve, ingesting only marginal amounts that are barely above what mainstream medicine considers a deficiency. True, the normal intake of vitamin B1 might be sufficient to prevent beriberi, but is it enough to prevent a learning disability or heart disease? As you'll learn later on, giving B1 supplements to children whose scores are low can increase their capacity to learn by 25 per cent. Nevertheless, medical orthodoxy won't even consider the possibility that the inability to concentrate could in fact be a symptom of a suboptimum vitamin B1 level.

THE REFINING PREDICAMENT

Perhaps most detrimental of all is the practice of refining our food. In this process, the whole food is separated into component parts, thereby discarding some of its nutrient-rich components. Refining is our most threatening food process because more and more of us are its victims. The percentage of our diet that comes from refined foods is at an all-time high, and by an ever-increasing margin.

Foods that nourish the animal kingdom share a remarkable characteristic: They all contain the vitamins, minerals, and accessory factors necessary for the one who eats them to metabolize and utilize them fully. Nature does not require us to forage for a second food in order to extract the nutritional value from the first food. In other words, partitioning food and discarding the nutrients necessary to metabolize the part of the food you do eat creates a nutrients shortage, forcing you to take in other foods to get those nutrient, thereby draining your reserves of those nutrients. In that way, the refining process turns foods into anti-nutrients – into foods that not only do not nourish us, but rob us of our already stored nutrient reserves which we need to remain healthy.

RICE

The first documented example of the harm wrought by refining is in the polishing of rice. Historically, the highly nutritious rice husk (or polishing) were discarded in making white rice, the nutritional staple of so many oriental cultures. A plethora of 'white rice only' diets produced an epidemic of beriberi that could be dramatically cured by a small quantity of rice polishings. Thus, the negative effects of refining nutrients out of foods was established and has proven just how essential those nutrients are.

SUGAR

The quintessential anti-nutrient is sugar. It is 100 per cent carbohydrate and therefore contains no vitamins or minerals. Nevertheless it needs to be metabolized instantly. The stores of all the nutrients involved in processing its constituent sugars, glucose and fructose are depleted in this process. As a result, these nutrients must be supplied from other dietary sources. Corn syrup, a simple sugar, rapidly increasing in usage, poses the same problem. To cite just one example, the critical glucose-metabolizing mineral chromium is severely depleted by consuming either sweetener.

REFINED WHEAT FLOUR

Refined flour (maida) is a close second to sugar and corn syrup in health threatening effects. However, its negative effect is more significant. While unmilled whole grains are indeed a significant source of essential minerals and other micronutrients, the milling process removes some 70-90 percent of these nutrients, leading to the same anti-nutrient effect ascribed to sugar. 'Enriching' the grains by adding an incomplete array of synthetic B vitamins and inorganic iron does little to change the results. The vital minerals – selenium, chromium, magnesium, zinc, manganese, and copper are not replaced, nor are key nutrients like essential fatty acids and B6. Yet the preachers of the food pyramid make no effort whatsoever to distinguish between whole grains and white flour, even though all nutritionists on the advisory panels are totally aware of the enormous nutritional depletion involved in the refining process. Worst of all, people are now consuming carbohydrates like pasta, cereal, bread, and crackers more than ever before, mistakenly believing they are making a healthy choice.

Many other factors combine to jeopardize our nutritional health. The environment, pollution, pesticides, petrochemicals, electronic emanations from our contemporary technology – all increase our need for nutrients that, by acting as antioxidants, are necessary to detoxify our systems from this chemical burden. The widespread use of antibiotics has created a generation of children with shortages of beneficial bacteria that help keep pathogenic yeast in check.

WARNING SIGNS OF DIETARY PROBLEMS

There are several symptoms that may indicate an excessively wrong diet or an overly malnourished condition. These signs are very important and require immediate attention if they occur at any time during childhood. Parents should suspect an overly under or mal-nourished condition if children display any of the following signs. Remember your child can be eating well in terms of quantity and still be lacking nutrients to be healthy.

1. Constant hunger or desire to eat.
2. Screaming or whining. A cheerful and joyful child is a sign of good health. When a child screams or whines without reason, it is often a sign imbalanced blood chemistry effecting the overall behaviour.
3. Tightness, lack of flexibility, or lack of motion.
4. Loss of the ability to crawl or walk.
5. Development of bow legs, as in rickets.
6. Failure to grow. If a child is small at birth, for example – 2-3 kilos, it is not necessarily a cause for concern. Smaller babies often have more vitality and capacity for growth than oversized babies. After birth, however, children normally grow very rapidly. Too much salt can inhibit growth and cause children to remain small and contracted.
7. Poor circulation. Salt can cause the peripheral capillaries to contract and inhibit blood flow. Cold hands or feet, or a pale colour may indicate this problem.
8. Abnormal weight. There is no fixed rate at which children gain weight. The standard height and weight charts that are commonly used today are often unreliable. The growth rates on

these charts tend to reflect averages among formula fed children. Normal ranges for breast-fed children have not yet been developed. Some children gain weight more rapidly, others more slowly. Babies who are smaller at birth tend to gain more rapidly, while larger infants tend to gain more slowly. As children get older, their rate of physical growth tends to slow down before adolescence.

As long as children have good appetites, parents need not be overly concerned about their weight. If children become abnormally thin or fat, however, it may be a sign of incorrect eating habits and be a sign for making changes in their daily diet. An excessive intake of salty snacks can cause a child to contract and become tight and skinny. In some cases, it can cause a child to retain water, fat, and to become overweight. Excessive sugar will cause yeast infections, cheek discolouration, worms in the stomach, and lowered immunity.

9. Dry or rough skin. Children normally have soft and smooth skin.
10. A change in bowel movement towards dark or hard stools. Bowel movement is one of the most important things to check when trying to determine whether your child's condition is healthy and he has a strong immune system. Colour and consistency are the two main factors to consider. A soft, yellow bowel movement is best for nursing infants. As children get older, the bowel movement normally becomes more yellowish-brown and firmer in consistency. If children have frequent green and watery stools, their condition is chronically out of balance. A child who eats good nourishing food normally has one bowel movement per day. The stools of such children do not have an unpleasant odour.
11. Irregular appetite. Fried, salty, and sugary foods can cause children to eat excessive amounts of food. Conversely, they can also cause the appetite to diminish because of their harmful effect on the digestive organs.

SCOURGE ONE OF TWENTY FIRST CENTURY: CHILDHOOD OBESITY

WHO has described obesity as a pandemic of the twenty first century. International authorities say that their fight against obesity (now defined as a medical problem) must be multidisciplinary in terms of behaviour, physical activity and most importantly food. Also, the control must start at an early age.

CHILDHOOD OBESITY AND ITS CONSEQUENCES

Previously, obesity was a problem for adults. Today this complicated condition is gaining prevalence in younger people. Obesity in childhood compromises the health of babies. More cases of diseases such as type 2 diabetes, high cholesterol, and hypertension are being diagnosed amongst the young. Apart from this, children may develop psychological problems due to frequent teasing, bullying, or rejection by their peers. This often leads to children having low self-esteem. Teens are marginalized by the way they look which can generate disorders such as bulimia, anorexia, depression, and lead to extreme habits like drug use and other harmful substances.

Bad habits learned in childhood can lead a child to suffer consequences of concern, mainly for their health. The risk of developing disorders during adolescence is a clear example of what can happen if the obese child does not receive adequate treatment and care regarding his diet and lifestyle.

Obese children are more likely to have:

1. Problems with bones and joints.
2. Difficulty in developing a sport or other physical exercise because of shortness of breath and fatigue.
3. Sleep disturbances, insomnia, sleep apnoea.
4. Premature maturity. Obese girls may start menstruating before puberty, develop irregular menstrual cycles or are late in starting.
5. High blood pressure, cholesterol, and cardiovascular disease.
6. Deranged liver.
7. Low morale, fatigue, and depression.
8. Low self-esteem, social isolation, discrimination.
9. Skin problems.
10. High sugar levels leading to diabetes.
11. Anorexia nervosa or bulimia.

In the opinion of experts, if obesity occurs during childhood and persists into adolescence without being treated, it will most likely be a permanent problem of adulthood and reduce life expectancy by upto 10 years.

WHAT IS THE CAUSE OF CHILDHOOD OBESITY?

1. Changing food patterns and modern day living. These are the main triggers in the rise of obesity. For many parents divided between multiple tasks, work and house management, it is more convenient to provide a quick meal for their children. The day starts with bread and jam before school, taking poories and paranthas in tiffin or buying snacks in the school canteen. Lunch is a cold meal and dinner is a home delivered pizza or burger from their favourite burger joint. Compound this with enough colas, chocolates, salty snacks, pastries, and ice creams along with 2 minute noodles or macaroni and you have the perfect recipe for an overweight child.

Followed day after day, these foods become a habit and children get used to eating food attractive in appearance but not containing nutrients or vital elements necessary for children to grow strong and healthy. Even in households with one parent working and the other staying back to look after the child, the most important thing is to satisfy the hunger of their children without worrying about nutrition or even the fact that they are compromising with the future of their child's health.

Just like many grandparents, new age parents are exaggeratedly concerned with the amount of food consumed by their children. They offer a menu without considering any control on fats, sugars, or salt. Gradually this scenario worsens and then they lament about their child not eating anything healthy or that the child is frequently ill. On the advice of their child specialist and food charts including the food pyramids, parents understand that their child's diet should be half carbohydrates, one third fats, and the rest proteins, but instead of eating whole wheat, brown rice, or vegetables, the kids are eating candy, soft drinks, and ice creams.

2. Sedentary Children. The lifestyle of children over the last decade has changed drastically. Most of their activities are concentrated around the television, computer, and video games. Many families lack the time, or find it inconvenient to make field trips, play outdoor games, and sports. Parents find it more convenient to leave their children in front of the television all afternoon rather than taking them to the park for some physical activity.

When asked from 100 parents about their kids activities, 95 per cent mentioned an average of 2 ½ hours in front of the television, computer, or video games, and the rest on tuitions and homework. This replacement of physical exercise by sedentary activities has led to an increasing number of children becoming obese, dull and lethargic.

3. Heredity. One of the main reasons for childhood obesity is the hereditary lifestyle. Parents pass on to their children genes which determine their height, colour of hair, eyes, etc., and they also pass on their eating habits. When heart disease, diabetes, or obesity is present in the parents, then the same eating patterns which led to their problems is followed by children.

Parents feel that childhood is the age to enjoy food. True, but food does not mean chips, pizzas, burgers, cookies, chocolates, and colas, and noodles. These are anti-foods with zero nutrition values. These can fill the stomach but cannot nourish the body nor lead to good growth and immunity. Following a diet of paranthas in the morning, fatty snacks, high sugar foods, mono diets of only potatoes and paneer will clog up the system and reduce the metabolic rate leading to weight gain and obesity.

4. Other factors. There are many other factors effecting childhood obesity including social influences, physiological changes, metabolic, and genetic disorders. Psychological disorders can be responsible for excessive overeating and weight gain.

5 SURE FIRE WAYS TO CONQUER CHILDHOOD OBESITY

There is an ongoing race to achieve the perfect therapy for treatment of obesity. Over the years, after studying and analyzing the success and failure of hundreds of treatments we have discovered the one best for children. It is a comprehensive approach that has given amazing results to 99.99 per cent of the children coming to us for weight reduction. This system has not only reduced their body mass, but has also given them a better physical shape, positive mental perception, confidence, and above all they have acquired healthy eating habits.

1. YOU WILL NEED TO TAKE 3 KEY POINTS FOR PERMANENT RESULTS

a) *Nutrition:* Teach them to eat well without restricting the quantities of meals. Putting limits on amount of food is a big error for growing children.

b) *Exercise:* Getting your kids to get involved in physical activity of their choice and having fun.

c) *Psychology:* Overweight children often have problems like distorted body perception, emotional need for food and other self-esteem issues. They need to be counseled with love and patience.

2. PARENT PARTICIPATION

A responsible parent invests time in the health of the child. They have a dual role of a teacher and a role model. Talking to kids about better foods or how important breakfast is for their immunity is one side of the coin. The other side involves the parent to be geared up for eating well himself and maintaining good health. They also require good skills for talking to children and knowing how to treat them. When children watch and observe their parents being careful about food and exercising regularly they will follow the same routines and the lifestyle inherited will be of good health.

3. SOCIAL ISSUES

Children can suffer abuse at the school, which undoubtedly provokes self-esteem to the point that they suffer anxiety or even depression. Some children might resort to binge eating while many have been known to vomit after eating. These food disorders can and should be avoided by helping the children and understanding their behaviour in school. Your child's behaviour at the locality park, with his neighbourhood friends and classmates should be observed.

You will be in a good position to assist them in developing confidence amongst peers. They should never have the feeling of diffidence or insecurity of being the class bumbler. This will ensure a correct body image and a feel good factor about themselves.

4. NO DIETING

We never advocate dieting for children and believe that neither should parents. Dietary regimes are too constrictive and evoke a feeling of denial in the person. Diets are usually followed for a few days and then older foods are reintroduced. This creates a yo-yo effect and is nothing but playing with the body.

The goal of weight reduction should not be only about thinning, but to learn about eating habits and healthy lifestyles. Nutritional guidelines must be tailored to their age without resorting to blind calorie reduction, especially in growing children. True and permanent weight reduction comes from applying correct nutritional foods which can raise the body's metabolic rate. Consistently eating natural, whole foods according to the orthomolecular way will give an excellent effect.

5. NUTRI-EDUCATION

You might manage to feed your children healthy food at home, but what about when they go out. Children are exposed to a variety of foods at school canteens, birthday parties; stay over at a friend and even at shopping trips. Parents often do not know what their child eats outside.

Children are not aware of what they are doing wrong. It is important that you impart nutrition education to your children. You must teach them to eat well themselves and not punish, scold, or nag about their food choices. They must learn what is healthy and what is not.

It will be in his favour to know how to recognize good food choices. They must agree and understand why the junk is called junk. The biggest lesson you can teach them is how to say no to foods that are not healthy for them. They should be able to do so with confidence when with friends or colleagues.

Finally change the home environment. If the refrigerator is full of sweets, chocolates, sugary drinks and the cupboard is full of noodles, biscuits, and bakery products, then these will remain an attraction for anyone in the house. When you don't get zero foods in the house, they will not be consumed. Having an open access to television and snacks all the time will make it very difficult for young obese children to change and regain a healthy weight.

SCOURGE TWO OF TWENTY FIRST CENTURY: ANAEMIC KIDS

Anaemia, one of the most common blood disorders, occurs when the level of healthy red blood cells (RBCs) in the body becomes too low. This can lead to health problems because RBCs contain haemoglobin, which carries oxygen to the body's tissues. Anaemia can cause a variety of complications, including fatigue and stress on bodily organs.

Anaemia can be caused by many things, but the three main bodily mechanisms that produce it are:

1. Excessive destruction of RBC's.
2. Blood loss.
3. Inadequate production of RBC's.

Among many other causes, anaemia due to nutritional problems (lack of iron, folic acid, or vitamin B12) is the leading complaint of many parents.

To understand anaemia, it helps to start with breathing. The oxygen we inhale doesn't just stop in our lungs. It's needed throughout our bodies to fuel the brain and all our other organs and tissues that allow us to function. Oxygen travels to these organs through the bloodstream — specifically in the red blood cells.

Red blood cells, or RBCs, are manufactured in the body's bone marrow and act like boats, ferrying oxygen throughout the rivers of the bloodstream. RBCs contain haemoglobin, a protein that holds onto oxygen. To make enough haemoglobin, the body needs to have plenty of iron. We get this iron, along with the other nutrients necessary to make red blood cells, from food.

WHAT ARE THE SYMPTOMS?

It's easy for people to overlook the symptoms of anaemia because it often happens gradually over time. Looking pale can be a sign of anaemia because fewer red blood cells are flowing through the blood vessels. The heart will beat faster in an effort to pump the same amount of blood and oxygen to the body, so the pulse may be faster than normal.

Anaemia can make children feel tired, weak, and cranky. It can cause pale skin, headaches, and a poor appetite. Kids with anaemia tend to get sick more often. Their brains and muscles are also affected.

As anaemia progresses, a child may feel short of breath, especially when climbing stairs, playing games, or working out. Iron deficiency, which occurs before iron deficiency anaemia develops, may affect a child's ability to concentrate, learn, and remember.

Prolonged or severe anaemia can cause marked irritability, decreased appetite, and slowed growth. In very severe cases, children can even go into heart failure. Anaemia is not contagious, so one cannot catch it from someone who has it.

WHY DO INFANTS GET ANAEMIC?

Infants who drink cow's milk in the first year of life are at risk for iron deficiency anaemia. Cow's milk does not have enough of the iron infants need to grow and develop and it is the most common dietary cause of iron deficiency in infants. Do not give cow's milk to your infant in the first year of life. Breastfed infants who do not eat iron-rich foods after the sixth month of life are also at risk of iron deficiency anaemia.

Toddlers (12 - 24 months of age) who drink a lot of cow's milk, have a diet low in iron, or already had iron deficiency as an infant are also at risk. If you use iron-fortified formula, do not give your child vitamin drops with iron. This combination provides too much iron and is not healthy. Stopping to breastfeed before your infant is 12 months of age is not recommended by most paediatricians.

After your child is 12 months old, if you stop breastfeeding, you should feed your toddler meat, chicken, fish, whole grains, enriched bread and cereal, dark green vegetables, and beans. Vitamin C is also important because it helps the body absorb iron. You should limit your child to less than 24 oz of cow's milk per day. (That's 3 cups of milk.) You might try giving your child yoghurt. Also ask your doctor if you should give your child vitamins with iron.

Iron deficiency anaemia can cause your infant or toddler to have mental, motor, or behavioural problems. These problems can be long lasting even after treatment cures the anaemia.

WHY DO CHILDREN GET ANAEMIC?

There are many, many reasons a child might become anaemic. The most common reason for a child to be anaemic is an inadequate supply of iron. Iron is a mineral that your body needs in order to make red blood cells. Children who lack enough iron will make small, pale, ineffective red blood cells.

Low levels of other nutrients, such as folic acid, can also cause anaemia. Many viral illnesses will cause brief anaemia in otherwise healthy children. Some children have red blood cells that are fragile and easily broken. This often occurs in hereditary conditions.

Some children have anaemia from blood loss. This can either be obvious blood loss, or long term, low grade blood loss, perhaps in the stool. A cow's milk allergy, for instance, is a common cause of hidden blood loss. Exposure to toxins, such as lead, can also cause anaemia.

WHY DO TEENS GET ANAEMIC?

Because teens go through rapid growth spurts, they can be at risk of iron deficiency anaemia. During a growth spurt, the body has a greater need for all types of nutrients, including iron, which we need to get in the foods we eat.

After puberty, girls are at more risk of iron deficiency anaemia than boys are. That's because a girl needs more iron to compensate for the blood loss during her menstrual periods. Also, a teen on a diet to lose weight may be getting even less iron.

Vegetarians are more at risk of iron deficiency anaemia than people who eat meat. Red meat is a rich source of iron.

HOW IS ANAEMIA TREATED?

The treatment of anaemia depends on what's causing it. Your paediatrician may get a blood test done to find the reason. If the anaemia is caused by iron deficiency, then foods rich in iron content and other nutrients should be added to the daily diet and must be supplemented with an iron supplement to be taken several times a day.

You may do a blood test after you have been on iron rich foods and the supplement. Even if the tests show that the anaemia has improved, the child may have to continue taking these foods for several months to replenish the body's total iron stores.

Because some children become nauseated if they take an iron supplement on an empty stomach, it can help to take it with food. Vitamin C boosts iron absorption, so eating lemon or amla during the meal will be a good idea. You can increase the chances that the iron your children gets from food will be absorbed by their body in other ways, too. For example, avoid serving tea with food because a substance in tea called tannin reduces the body's ability to absorb iron found in the food or iron supplement. Milk can also interfere with iron absorption, so don't pair milk with iron-rich foods if you are concerned about them getting enough iron.

Some people need more iron than others. Girls need more than guys, for example. And a girl who has heavy periods has a greater need for iron than a girl who has a light flow.

There are other nutritional reasons why someone's body may not make enough RBCs. Vitamin B12 and folic acid are also needed to make red blood cells, so it's important to get enough of these nutrients in their diet. If the bone marrow is not working properly because of an infection, blood loss due to an injury, chronic illness, or certain medications, anaemia can develop. If your child's anaemia is caused by another medical condition, doctors will work to treat the cause. People with some types of anaemia will need to see a specialist, called a haematologist, who can provide the right medical care for their needs. The good news is that most cases of children's anaemia are easily treated. And in a few weeks they'll have their energy back!

To make sure your children get enough iron, folic acid and vitamin B12, give then a nutrient rich diet every day.

SHOULD MY CHILD BE TESTED FOR IRON DEFICIENCY?

If you're worried and think your child might have nutritional anaemia, talk to your paediatrician. Infants at risk of iron deficiency should be checked with a blood test at 9-12 months of age. Toddlers should be checked 6 months later and at 24 months.

PREVENTING ANAEMIA IN YOUR CHILD

The first step in preventing anaemia in children is to ensure breastfeeding for the first 12 months when the baby is born. In case of artificial feeding, use safe iron supplements prescribed by your doctor.

Thereafter for whole life, you can control anaemia with proper food given to them. A nutritionally sound diet balanced in all nutrients and given to maximize its benefits is the essential foundation for good growth and development.

Another important measure is to rule out the presence of intestinal worms and parasites. Often children can be infected with worms and show all or some of the signs like anal itching, grinding of teeth, voracious appetite, constant nose digging, irritability, and convulsions. Safe deworming can be done naturally and with homoeopathic remedies. You must ensure that children wash their hands after going to poop, playing in the mud, and before eating with their hands.

The entire exercise of de-worming can come to naught without taking these cares since the larvae of the worms are present under the nails. The same going into the mouth will re-infect the child and a vicious cycle can start.

FOODS TO PREVENT ANAEMIA

All your focus should be on presenting a good, varied diet with adequate nutrition. Nutritional anaemia can be prevented by including foods such as meat, chicken, fish, egg yolk, beans, lentils, chickpeas, soybeans, peas, spinach, broccoli, cauliflower, beetroot, dark green leaves, mangoes, and grapes.

As important as it is to feed your child these foods, it is equally vital that they are properly combined to increase absorption of nutrients. Random mixing of nutrient rich foods can do more harm by inhibiting nutrition absorption. And you will be left wondering why your child suffers when you feed him the best foods.

The foods given in the '12 week incredible immunity plan' are rich in macronutrients and micronutrients including iron, folic acid, and vitamin B12. Following this pattern of feeding can increase the haemoglobin level in the blood since all the above foods are included in the plan. They are also mixed in a way to extract maximum benefit from them.

3 FROM 'YUCK' TO 'WOW'

A child refusing to eat is a common complaint of many parents. And oh! How often. It is a situation that is rightly called a 'no-win confrontation', that is to say, a hopeless struggle to win. How does one get out of this impasse?

Dining is diverse and complicated enough already. It requires time, money, and a little expertise. As a parent you have to invest yourself and if you have a passive attitude to food, it will be difficult. When you let yourself be carried away by the whirlwind of time and a fast paced life, then sandwiches, pizzas, quiches, and snacks are the only foods you will be serving as meals.

Also if you have grown up in a family where going to the market to buy fruits and vegetables is a chore given to the cooks, and meals are only considered as a response to a biological need, 'we eat to live', then you might have to work harder. Hurrying to make food 'practical', 'fast', and trying to avoid the kitchen are not going to get your kids to eat healthy, or even make them appreciative of how closely food is connected to the upkeep of the body.

Families where the most valued rewards are intellectual usually struggle to invest time and money in food. Historically, culturally in intellectual circles, food is secondary. One gets to hear from family members, "We did not attach much importance because there are other ways to be rewarded and be happy." Ironically families like these are unhappy about their health, and members suffer from gastritis, acidity, ulcers, high blood pressure, diabetes, and can be overweight or underweight besides complaining of constipation, haemorrhoids, and piles.

NO, IT IS NOT MISSION IMPOSSIBLE TO CHANGE!

To permanently change the way we eat, you must take into account the lifestyle, tastes, and culture of your family. That's why diets are not sustainable for long. For the sake of thinness, we might accept drastic changes, difficult as they might be sometimes with the feeling that it is easier to deny ourselves for a short time. But such endeavours are headed towards failure and we bounce right back to our old ways of eating without any regards to nutrition or health.

Since it is the lifestyle that must reflect good eating practices, let's look at how the children get bad habits and who is responsible.

EATING SUGAR VS PAPAYA

A few years ago, both the authors had gone out to dine at a restaurant. It had been an engrossing day with the usual cases of parents complaining that their child didn't like fruits, or had no taste for vegetables. At a table close to ours sat a young couple with an infant in the mother's arms whom she was feeding lovingly from a bowl on the table. To my co-author's surprise the child was being fed 'Rasgulla and its syrup' (a highly sweetened delicacy made with cottage cheese). Unable to restrain herself, my co-author went up to their table and requested to sit with them. They were quite surprised but looking at her dignified attire and politeness, they welcomed her. She asked the child's age which the mother mentioned to be 5 months. 5 months!! Aghast at the tender age, she pointed out to the mother that till the age of 12 months, a child's taste buds are still developing. Even after that for the next few years her tongue will be acquiring new experiences and registering them in her brain.

If the mother continues to do as she is doing now, soon she will be running after the child with food to eat and the child will find all good foods bland and tasteless. There was no way that the sweetness of an apple, or an orange, or a carrot could compare with the concentrated sugar syrup. The child will only want biscuits, sweets, candy, chocolates, ice creams, colas, and the like. Fortunately the parents understood their error and thanked her for her advice.

EXPERIMENT ONE

Try this at home with your child or even yourself to experience the effect of sugar on the tongue and the message it sends to the brain. Take 2 teaspoons of sugar and eat them followed by a bowl of papaya. We are certain that you will not only find it hard to eat the full bowl of fruit, you might even find the papaya repulsive, comment that it has a bad odour, that it is tasteless, and you feel like vomiting.

If your child has ever said these things for papaya, now you know who is responsible. A high sugar diet perverts the sense of taste at any age. It prevents children from exploring new tastes, textures, and flavours. It keeps the body addicted to sugary snacks and zero nutrition foods since each time the tongue requires the same taste, the sweetness, and everything else seems totally bland in comparison.

FRUIT COLOURS-VS-PACKED FOODS

Most parents take their children to malls and shopping centers and very rarely to the vegetable and fruit market. At the mall, our eyes are enamoured by the array of rainbow colours. In fact, the human eye finds it highly pleasing to view things in colour. It gives us a sense of beauty and attraction.

The packaging food industry has done its research extremely well in this field. They have tested different colours for their products to get the maximum eyeballs. You will find that many of the processed foods are attractively packaged in bright reds, greens, and yellows. Chips and biscuits, cornflakes and soup packets are all designed to woo the customer and attract the kids. Cartoon figures on the boxes and soft toys given after meals are strategies to bring in children with their parents.

EXPERIMENT TWO

Try this at home with your children to see how well they choose. Make two baskets, fill one with colourful packs of chocolates, chips, and cookies. Fill the other with deep red apples, green pears, bananas, black grapes, stripped melons, strawberries, raspberries, and cherries. Bring your child in front of the baskets and observe which one he goes towards. 95 per cent of urban children head straight for the cookies and chocolates, and reach to grab them. Only 5 per cent head towards the fruit basket. With your child's decision, you will know who's responsible.

It is human nature to be dazzled by colours. Nature has provided us fruits and vegetables in a rainbow of colours for a reason. They are not dull black and white, and neither are they of only green colour. You have red, golden and green apples, yellow and purple bananas, red and lime green pears, red and yellow mangoes, pink litchis, brown chikkoos, black, pink and green grapes besides the pomegranates, oranges, kinnoos, sweet limes, water melons, cantaloups, kiwis, and plenty more for a reason.

Nature has provided red, yellow and green bell peppers, brown potatoes, red and white radishes, purple aubergines, red tomatoes, orange and pink carrots, and many more to attract the human eye.

Man has aped nature to market his dead foods and feed the new generation. The only real loser is parents and children themselves. Your child's choice of multicoloured packs gives him zero nutrition, addictive spices, artificial colours, additives, preservatives, flavour enhancers, and more chemicals.

His correct choice of fruits will give him nourishment, real flavours, natural aroma, wholesome taste, and build his immunity, improve growth, increase his brain power, and boost his strength and stamina. The choice you want your child to make lies in your hands – the parents.

STAGES OF CHILD'S GROWTH VIS A VIS FOOD AND TASTE

FIRST STAGE (0 TO 12 MONTHS)

This is the easiest stage for parents. The child will drink mother's milk and after few months will develop taste for newer foods like puree of fruits, vegetables, cereals, etc – all fed and controlled by the mother. At this stage, the child cares little for taste, or any favourite foods. If the mother is aware of health building foods and builds her child's taste buds to like these then she would have laid the foundation of health for her child.

SECOND STAGE (1 YEAR TO 3 YEARS)

At this stage the child has started forming fixed ideas of taste and may refuse foods he does not relish. He will be attracted to bright colours and if these are of packed foods then he will always be seeking more of them. At this stage he may expand his choices to include foods resembling his favourite ones. His main criterion for making a choice is taste only.

THIRD STAGE (3 YEARS TO 12 YEARS)

Children in the middle years are in a stage of transition from toddlers to teenagers. They change from being completely dependent upon their parents to being more independent. They develop a longer span of concentration, more fluent speech, greater physical agility and control, the ability to reflect about themselves and their actions, and to regulate their emotions and behaviour. Their thinking becomes deeper, involving larger areas of the brain than in early childhood, and they begin seeking explanations for many of the things they see around them.

The child becomes more aware of foods and recognizes that he will always have a choice to make. He can be moulded to newer types of dishes and may try all of them if brought up well in the last two stages. Parents can nurture the seed of good healthy eating planted years ago and experience joy from watching their child grow healthy and strong.

The child can be taught to explore new foods and derive fun and excitement from the process. He can be moulded to experiment with different tastes, flavours, textures, and be flexible with food options. The criterion will still be taste but the practice of trying new foods and constantly growing in food choices will be built at this stage.

FOURTH STAGE (12 YEARS TO 19 YEARS)

As children enter the teen years, they are exposed to many outside influences and begin comparing them with the attitudes, dreams, and patterns of daily life that they have observed at home. They become increasingly sensitive to the way in which others see them. They will be associating with teachers, playmates, and friends, and their scope of interaction continues to widen. They become interested in the outside world and their relationships to it, and are more keenly aware of male and female differences. At this stage they will be actively asking, or refusing certain foods. If parents have done their job right, then at this stage education about the relationship of food to good health can be imparted.

The child can be shown how her choices will affect her looks, body weight, skin, hair, and physique. She realizes the importance of eating nourishing food and learns about which foods to avoid completely. She is conscious of food and its effect on her body and beauty. During the late teen years, children will stop eating foods for taste alone. They will pick and choose food for building muscles, reducing and maintaining weight, glowing complexion, better academic performance, and for sports reasons.

FIFTH STAGE (19 YEARS TO 21 YEARS)

As physical growth slows down, a child's mental development accelerates. The latter part of teen years are ideal for learning, study, and the development of intellectual and artistic abilities, as well as for the development of physical strength and coordination. During this stage and thereafter children will remain actively involved in reading, writing, mathematics, cooking, music, art, sports, and other activities that challenge them mentally and physically.

He raises his own awareness through books, internet, television, and peers. A full amalgamation of eating for health and taste can be done. He now has the capacity to imbibe health as a lifestyle. He will educate himself on how healthy, wholesome foods can be made into delicious meals. Parents can congratulate themselves if their child remains focused on the nutrient aspects of food.

This stage completes the full cycle of food and taste with real visible results of optimal fitness, proper food combining, and an individual that has taken control of his own life and family.

The adult entering the world has taken the base learning that food must serve the body – healthy food can be made tasty and real pleasure comes from eating food that looks appealing, has an inviting aroma, is pleasing to the tongue and most of all is beneficial for the body.

5 SECRETS OF GETTING YOUR KIDS TO LOVE WHAT YOU MAKE

As a parent you are responsible for what your child eats and not your child. Left to the child, he will want to eat only junk foods since he loves their taste. But you cannot raise your hands and say my child does not eat anything. You will have to work a little hard and convert your finicky, fussy eaters to love what you make for them.

If your children do not want to go to school, we are certain you will be tough on them and pack them off to class. Then why give up when they want only ice cream, or chips, or noodles.

FLEXIBILITY

It is important that parents provide a balanced and varied diet but never impose. Vegetables, fruit, meat, fish, whole grains, etc. are to be introduced gradually without hurting the taste of the child, without forcing, by accepting any refusal and trying a new format a few days later. Avoid falling into the routine of making the same recipes again and again if the child has not liked the same first time. Be flexible and make the time to eat fun for yourself and your children.

Be flexible about being rigid also. Many children are willingly content with the same menu every day. Once the child has liked some food and it is balanced meal, there is no reason to oppose the child's desire. He has his whole life ahead of him to become a gourmet! You won't run out of ideas once you introduce the '12 week incredible immunity plan' in his lifestyle.

NO STRESS

To get children to taste new foods you must avoid stress in their schedules. Prepare tasty dishes and offer them in a nice and relaxed family atmosphere. A meal with parents whose gaze is riveted on the screen of the television is not very inviting for a child of 8 or 15 months who requires an emotional exchange. Watching parents eat while looking at the news at night gives the child the feeling that he must do the same. He will grow up to eat while watching his favourite shows without any interest in the food. If you feel that television is your best distraction to get him to eat, then you are wrong on several counts.

Organizing a picnic on the weekend is an original idea for introducing new foods to your children. Similarly, make the meal at home and serve it 'cafe style' – course after course. This is a very popular method with kids. Give them some snacks to start with and follow with main course. Let there be no mistake: There is no question of changing family patterns, definitely go on a picnic for lunch, or prepare new dishes for children but always keeping their health as top priority. This is done only to give the child a taste for eating, to show that the 'dining table' is for pleasure and not a boxing ring.

A LITTLE COMMON SENSE

Eating time must be undramatic and regarded with lucidity, and good sense. In our society, frequency of eating is far more than is necessary. The daily intakes of individuals can sometimes be almost 20 to 50 per cent higher than the theoretical needs.

Parents may feel that their child does not eat enough, eat often enough, or eat substantial portions. But the evidence shows that these views of parents are fundamentally flawed. Furthermore, each child has his own individual needs and can never be compared with general theoretical standards. The differences between large and small eaters can vary from simple to double. There are normal children who eat a lot and normal children who eat little. Some children do very well with 1-2 good meals a day, and express their boredom with slow chewing when forced to eat more. There is no scientific reason to force children to eat 3 times a day if they do not want. In any case they will be changing to this social rule at one time or another as they grow up. So it's not worth making eating time an occasion of protracted conflict without result. Low dietary needs coupled with a good development and normal activities are evidence of good health.

NO HUNGER GAMES

As a parent you need to understand that remaining focused on the appetite of the child all the time – about what he eats and what he leaves is counterproductive. The key advice to parents here is that, under no pretext and in any circumstance they should force the child to eat. You must stop using force, fraud, games, etc.

Parents should also never talk to kids about food with disinterest. If the mother puts the plate before the child with anger and takes it back, still filled with rage, even without saying a word, it is doomed to fail. Similarly, if she told the child: "Here, take your food. You eat, you do not eat, I do not care. I will take your plate away in 10 minutes and you will have nothing else to eat here tonight" – the result will be automatic. The child will show stubbornness and not eat. A stubborn child is always stronger than his parents. Do not confront the child with ultimatums but use diplomacy.

COOK WITH LOVE

Children will be ready to change if they watched their parents cook and if the meals were a highlight of the day. The secret of children's kitchen is the pleasure that is passed onto the food. When one wants to give pleasure, it makes good food. You must cook what you love: Gather the right products, good ideas, and then make the food according to your child's taste! There is no need to complicate things, even simple things like sandwiches and milkshakes can be made utterly delicious when done right. Above all, the food must be simmered with love. Take away foods and fast food centers can never ever compete with this type of food. If the child realizes that his parents put less emphasis on making food, he will take less pleasure in eating that food.

2 SAMPLE CASES FROM MY NUTRITION CLINIC

CASE ONE

A young girl of 17 years came to me with her parents to consult for increasing her height. She had heard from her classmates the good results they were getting and one of her friends had gained 4 inches in a span of 8 months after eating my prescribed foods.

From appearance, she was a healthy girl with all the correct growth milestones having been achieved and without any history of disease. On asking about her food intake throughout the day she described the following:

Early morning: Parantha + Tea or Biscuits + Tea

Breakfast / Tiffin: Puffed rice + Papad + Chips + Chocolates (shared with friends)

Dosa + Ice cream or Khasta or Chola bhatura (eaten in the canteen)

Lunch: Rotis + Rice + Dal + Vegetables

Evening: Glass of milk

Dinner: Mutton/ Chicken/ Fish + Rotis + Rice

I was surprised that she was not eating anything substantial till the afternoon. Growing children need a nutritious breakfast while she was eating mostly from the school canteen. Her diet didn't have any fruits, raw vegetables (salads) or yoghurt. She was predominantly on a diet of junk and cereals with a smattering of proteins. Essential vitamins, minerals, and enzymes were markedly absent. Her water intake was minimal at five glasses which she took with meals to push the food down. It was no wonder that she was short and at age 17 still four feet eight inches.

I introduced her to newer foods, mostly from the foods given **in the '12 weeks incredible immunity plan'** and supplemented her diet with good quality multivitamins and essential oils. She was asked to exercise and do stretches in the evening. Soon her body started responding to the changed food patterns and there was a growth spurt that took her height to five feet one inch.

Here a little about canteen foods is worth mentioning. There have been numerous occasions when I have been invited to well known, reputed schools to address their students and have had an opportunity to look at their canteens and the foods served there.

The meals offered at school canteens should worry all parents. Hygiene of the products and facilities is the main concern not to talk of the nutritional aspect of the meals. The quality of ingredients and the hygiene maintained at these canteens is appalling.

Most of these canteens are given out on contract and run by managers who have little concern or knowledge of food preparation and how to maintain hygiene standards. Usually the back areas and store rooms are infested with rodents and cockroaches and the utensils used for cooking seem as if they have not been washed for months. These canteens are staffed by workers negligent about personal hygiene. You can often see them going to the toilet and coming back to knead the flour or chop the potatoes without washing their hands.

The canteen has a budget on which it is run. Their main goal remains the same: Find meals at cheapest price possible. The savings are the profit of the contractors. To offer competitive prices, some managers would offer dishes that appeal to children but certainly whose nutritional value is questionable. The bread, buns, rice, flour, and bakery products like patties, biscuits, etc. are of extremely poor quality. Profits are made at the expense of nutritional quality.

The question is whether it is possible to get a reasonably balanced meal at a school canteen without it being a food poisoning hazard. The answer is 'No'.

PARENTS SURVEYED

During our interactions with parents, nearly eight in ten parents say they are willing to pay more for better quality and safety of meals at school. But the foundation of good, healthy meals at schools can only be laid by following strict norms of safety and hygiene. There must be regular checks by the Municipal Committees and inspections by Health inspectors. Kitchens have to be designed as per rules and the menu served has to adhere to balanced nutrition for children.

CASE TWO

A harried and depressed mother came to me with her 10 year old son and complained that he just didn't eat anything. He got frequent colds and coughs and had a history of Primary Complex as an infant. She was worried that he was not growing at a good rate and all his classmates were taller and more robust than him. He didn't look his age and was often ridiculed by peers. He was most interested in computer games and television with absolutely no desire to participate in games or sports. On asking about his food intake throughout the day, she described the following:

Early morning: Tea or Milk

Breakfast / Tiffin: Namkeen mixtures + Biscuits or Bread-Jam (Roti + Vegetables sent were returned without being eaten)

Lunch: Rotis + Vegetables (only Potatoes or Lady finger)

Evening: Noodles or Macaroni or Bread + Jam or Halwa

Dinner: Pizza or Burgers or Poori with Potatoes or + Rice with Kidney beans

(He would demand for chocolates, biscuits, and cold drinks frequently.)

I was not surprised that the child had low immunity and was often sick. His diet was deprived of all nutrients and was totally on a sickness forming food habit. When young bodies are given foods made in the factory like cookies, namkeen mixtures, chips, chocolates, bread, jam, tea, noodles then the body is unable to extract anything for itself and starts to slow down. The excretory systems like lungs and colon clog up. The body will try to detox itself by throwing out mucous in form of cold and will be constipated.

The blood will be highly toxic with fried foods, and an only potato and lady finger diet. His tongue taste had got used to high salt, high sugar, and high spices.

I gradually introduced foods from the **'12 week incredible immunity plan'**. As his tongue taste started changing, he started relishing fruits. I balanced his diet with nutritious ice creams, biryanis, kebabs from **'Superfoods- Make Your Child a Genius'**. Within a few weeks his mother mentioned he was more energetic and had started playing at the neighbourhood park. After 6 months, the transformation was complete. In my last consultation with him, his mother said that he had not caught a cold when the season changed which was a first in his life. He had participated in a school dance and was making more friends due to improved health. Even his teachers felt that he had gained a new confidence.

Both the cases like thousands of others were converted to healthier eating only due to tasty foods introduced to them. Rich mixtures of fruits and nuts were a good substitute for their sugar intake. Their body chemistry changed with the balanced nutrition given to them throughout the day. And nearly all the children I have given these foods to loved them for their taste and flavours. You too can make your child love his food.

KEEPING THE JOY ALIVE IN YOUR COOKING

Vary the pleasures! Learn to vary the composition of the meals without making changes in their balanced nutrients. Respecting the contribution of each family of food, infinite meals can be prepared with numerous combinations of textures and flavours. Even the simple bottle gourd can be made in a different style every day for 15 days without repeating its look, aroma, and taste.

Cooking for your family should not be a chore, but sometimes it ends up feeling that way. You can change that by getting Dad and the kids in on making a meal. Set up a family night where everyone gets together and makes dinner together. The children decide the menu, both of you do the chopping and cooking, then back to the kids for garnishing and plating. It will save time and be less stressful, making mealtimes much more enjoyable for everyone.

There are many easy starter meals to begin with for bringing the children into the kitchen. Our Italian pizza night can be great hit with the family and so can making the Sunday breakfast. You can opt from Kebabs to Sandwiches, Frankies to Corn Chaats. Keep in mind that when it comes to 'life skills', cooking is a reality for everyone. So cooking with kids is something all parents should consider.

There are many things like warming up pre-made meals, garnishing, peeling fruits, etc. that are good activities for children to help in, and have some fun while doing it. Like when making the breads, the children can knead the dough. They can punch the air out of it and knead it again after it has risen, to give mom that extra moment of peace. The little ones especially get excited with these projects, squealing with delight when the bread rises and swelling with confidence when everyone in the house is told that they made the bread. Similarly with the salads, toppings, evening drinks, and snacks.

I know parents who said that their kids would be least interested in cooking but were amazed when the same children got hooked to sharing the work. They developed a keener sense of taste and visual appeal. Children will also eat more readily what they have made even if they are not happy with the outcome. Once you start getting them involved, you will observe the great fun your children will derive from making their food. There are many meals that don't involve cooking that you could start the kids off with, such as sandwiches, fruit mixtures, and salads. These types of meals are good for getting them used to how things work in the kitchen before they are ready to start cooking. We are not saying that your child should become a chef but cooking is a terrific confidence booster for children of any age. It makes them feel more useful around the house and they take greater pride in getting appreciated for the meals they do prepare.

Be sure to teach kitchen safety and the importance of supervision at all times. Discuss the meal and steps necessary with them before starting so that they have an idea of what they will need to do as well as an idea of how long it will take. This will help them enjoy the process more. Be patient with them. We know you will have to clean up the mess they will make in the beginning. So have a sink of soapy water to soak the dishes as they get done with them.

Food and cooking are intimate parts of daily life and the heart of most great family memories. So, have fun and start making lasting memories that could turn into lasting traditions for your family.

4 ENTER THE FOOD WARRIORS

ONE HUNDRED YEARS AGO

About a century back, beriberi was prevalent in eastern Asia, where rice is the staple food, and also in the Pacific islands and South America. It involves paralysis and numbness, starting from the legs leading to cardiac and respiratory disorders and finally death. In the Dutch East Indies soldiers, sailors, prisoners, mine workers, plantation workers, and persons admitted to a hospital for minor ailments were dying of the disease by the thousands. Young men in seemingly good health sometimes died suddenly, in terrible distress through an inability to breathe.

Then a young Dutch physician, Christian Eijkman, was asked by the Dutch government to study the disease. For 3 years he made little progress. One day, he noticed that the chickens in the laboratory chicken house were dying of a paralytic disease closely resembling beriberi. His studies of the chickens' disease were suddenly brought to an end, when the chickens that had not yet died recovered and no new cases developed. He found, on investigating the circumstances that the man in charge of the chickens had been feeding them, from 17 June to 27 November, on polished rice (with the husks removed) prepared in the military hospital kitchen for the hospital patients. Then a new cook took charge of the kitchen who refused, as Eijkman was to report in his address while accepting the Nobel Prize for physiology and medicine in 1929, to 'allow military rice to be taken for civilian chickens'. The disease had broken out among the chickens on 10 July and disappeared during the last days of November.

It was immediately confirmed that a diet of polished rice caused death of chickens in 3 or 4 weeks, whereas they remain in good health when fed unpolished rice. A study of 300,000 prisoners in 101 prisons in the Dutch East Indies was then made, and it was found that the incidence of beriberi was three hundred times as great in the prisons where polished rice was used as a staple diet as in those where unpolished rice was used. Eijkman found that he could isolate an extract from the bran of the rice that had protective power against beriberi. At first he thought that some substance in the bran acted as an antidote for a toxin assumed to be present in polished rice, but by 1907 he and his collaborator, Gerrit Grijns concluded that the bran contains a nutrient substance that is required for good health.

IMMUNITY ON THE PLATE!

From time immemorial man has sought the fountain of youth and health. There have been fables and folklores about a panacea which would give everlasting health. While these are myths written years ago, the scientific community has been working tirelessly to uncover the secrets behind keeping the body in perfect health. Surprisingly, the magic formula has not been found in cosmetic products or owned by plastic surgeons but hidden on your very own dinner plate.

Early indicators of atherosclerosis, the most common cause of heart disease, begins as early as childhood and adolescence. Atherosclerosis is related to high blood cholesterol levels, which are associated with poor dietary habits.

Osteoporosis, a disease where bones become fragile and can break easily, is associated with inadequate intake of calcium.

Type 2 diabetes, formerly known as adult onset diabetes, has become increasingly prevalent among children and adolescents as rates of overweight and obesity rise. Recent studies estimate that more children born after 2000 will develop diabetes in their lifetime.

Overweight and obesity, influenced by poor diet and inactivity, are significantly associated with an increased risk of diabetes, high blood pressure, high cholesterol, asthma, joint problems, and poor health status.

Advances made in food chemistry and its effects on the biochemistry of human body show that some foods actually contain micronutrients that slow the wearing out of our cells. The contents of your plate decide not only your health but also your longevity. The weight of the years can be reduced, your skin can look young and supple, your vital organs can function optimally for years, you can prevent diseases, and remain strong when you make it a habit to introduce these elixirs of fitness in your family's menu.

ALL THE GOOD STUFF

It is a consensus in the scientific field that a higher consumption of these healthy foods is associated with a reduced risk of myriad diseases and early aging. Scientists are now working on understanding exactly why 'nutrient dense' foods provide health protection, and they have identified many compounds present in these foods that appear to be critical for prevention of chronic diseases. Among the most researched are the antioxidants, polyphenols, phytoestrogens, omega – 3,6,9, dietary fibres and resistant starches concentrated in foods such as fruits, vegetables, whole grains, nuts, seeds, and legumes.

WHAT IS A 'NUTRIENT DENSE' FOOD?

Many foods have nutrients in them, but how much do you need to get the 'most' nutrients? This is what the concept nutrient dense addresses. Dense literally means 'massed closely together', and with respect to nutrients can be interpreted as – the most nutrient per amount or serving size.

ANTIOXIDANTS

The health-promoting effects of whole foods are thought to be partially related to their abundant and complex antioxidant profile. Nothing protects your health and extends life more than a steady supply of antioxidants to your cells. Food antioxidants are a huge extended family of chemical warriors that directly oppose oxygen charged molecules hell bent on damaging cells. Antioxidants are a major police force of the body helping to actively deflect virtually all chronic diseases and the aging process itself. A deficiency of the antioxidants can leave your child extremely vulnerable. Vitamins and minerals can double as antioxidants. So can enzymes and myriad exotic compounds that have been discovered to have biochemical activity. Free radicals and unstable oxygen species are known to promote the development of atherosclerosis, cancer, arthritis, diabetes, and a host of other conditions later in life.

It is also known that antioxidants can protect you from the damage these molecules produce in your cells, that different antioxidants provide protection to different parts of your body and cells, and that antioxidants work together as a team. Therefore, your child needs more than just a high amount of a single antioxidant, like vitamin C; she needs the gamut of antioxidants provided by a varied whole foods diet to keep the reactive oxygen species like free radicals 'in check', thus minimizing the damage they can cause.

POLYPHENOLS: THE SECRET OF YOUTH

These substances are considered the 'backbone' for most of the antioxidants found in plants. They exhibit characteristics like anti-inflammatory and antiseptic effects and are instrumental in combating oxidative stress.

1. Against cardiovascular disease: Polyphenols taken during a meal would fight against the oxidation of bad cholesterol. This would prevent the phenomena and the cause of the blockage of arteries.
2. Against cancer: Like all antioxidant compounds, polyphenols prevent the formation of tumours. In fact, they will even protect against harmful genetic mutations.

3. Against heavy metals: Polyphenolic compounds assist in detoxifying the body by chelating with metals and facilitating their removal.

PHYTOESTROGENS

Phytoestrogens, a special class of phyto-nutrients that include isoflavones and lignans, are found in plant-based foods such as flaxseeds, sesame, garlic, dried apricots, alfalfa sprouts, almonds, onion, watermelon, and berries. In the past few years, phytoestrogens have received recognition as yet another unique health-promoting feature offered by whole, natural, and nutritious foods. Subsequent experimental research has clearly shown that isoflavones are converted in the body to hormone-like compounds that have the ability to modulate oestrogen activity and dampen its potentially damaging effects in cells within the female reproductive organs.

OMEGA 3 AND 6: ESSENTIAL FATTY ACIDS

Free radicals are responsible for skin damage. They cause pimples, acne, wrinkles, loss of elasticity; and fragility of skin tissue. Essential fatty acids compensate for the assault of free radicals in the cell membrane structure and form a reserve for the cell. This contribution helps to provide structural elements necessary for the youth of the skin. Healthy skin is a sure sign of good health.

The brain is made up of upto 20 per cent essential fatty acids. These are the polyunsaturated fats which provide neuron membranes thickness and flexibility for optimal exchange of information. For proper brain functioning, these fatty acids (omega 3 and 6) need to be consumed in the correct proportion. Due to an imbalanced diet, their level decreases and as your child gets older, the risk of developing cognitive impairment increases. Studies published in 2003, show that people who consumed these oils had decreased their risk of suffering from Alzheimer's disease by 60 per cent and protected their brain's capacity for memory, logic, and reasoning.

Omega-3 fatty acids, one of the polyunsaturated fats are critical components of the membranes in every one of your cell, so they are absolutely vital to your body's ability to function properly. The parent omega-3 fatty acid, the one from which all others are made, is alpha-linolenic acid, and it is essential because your body can't make it, therefore, it must be obtained from your diet.

Omega-3 (ALA, EPA, DHA) besides playing a central role in cell membranes also participates in many biochemical processes in the body like the regulation of blood pressure, the elasticity of vessels, immune responses, anti-inflammatory aggregation of blood platelets, etc. Good permeability of cell membranes allows entry of nutrients into the cells and allows the waste produced by them to be eliminated.

Omega-6 (LA, GLA) is the other essential polyunsaturated fat which the body does not make on its own and hence requires a regular supply from the food. This crucial element has a role to play in the nervous system, cardiovascular balance, immunity, wound healing, allergic reactions, and inflammations.

DIETARY FIBRES AND RESISTANT STARCHES

In the large intestines, dietary fibre binds to carcinogens, excess hormones such as oestrogens, bile acids, and toxins like pesticides, promoting their excretion from the body. Dietary fibre also supports healthy digestion and, since it is the preferred food of the cells that make up the lining of the intestinal tract, is necessary for a healthy intestinal tract overall.

When your children eat whole grains, they get high levels of minerals, a range of vitamins including all the energy-supporting B vitamins, and the essential fats. When processed, a whole grain loses its bran, which contains most of its fibre, minerals, and B vitamins; and its germ, which contains its essential fats and the family of protective vitamin E compounds called the tocopherols. From refined grains in comparison, you get a large amount of simple carbohydrates and starch, a bit of protein, and only a few vitamins from a food that started out with thousands of healthy compounds and a full spectrum of vitamins.

Time and again, epidemiological studies – a type of study in which the diet consumed by individuals is compared to their development of disease over a period of years or decades – shows that people who consume these foods have a reduced risk of developing cardiovascular disease (CVD), arthritis, and cancer than people whose diets emphasize processed, refined un-whole foods. When your children start practicing wholesome eating, they will show a decreased rate of aging and diseases in comparison with those who do not.

VITAMINS A, C, E AND SELENIUM: BETTING ON THE WINNING QUARTET!

Carotenoids: Carotenoids are a group of phytonutrients that lend the red, orange, and yellow hues to fruits and vegetables. Carotenoids are present in all living organisms, but humans are not able to make them and must get them from food. Some carotenoids can be converted in your body to vitamin A; however, the reason carotenoids have received so much recent attention has more to do with their significant antioxidant effects. Several recent studies have shown an association between the consumption of foods rich in carotenoids and the lower risk of degenerative diseases, premature aging, and reduced effects of environmental pollution.

Carotenoids found in foods are varied, and over 60 different carotenoids have been identified. In humans, at least 8 of these have been shown to be absorbed and to have beneficial activities. Of these carotenoids, beta-carotene is the most recognized and talked about since the earliest studies on carotenoids found an association between high levels of beta-carotene consumption and a decrease in disorders. Of the varied carotenoids found in humans, lycopene is present in the blood in the highest concentration. Lycopene is found in tomatoes, watermelon, and papaya, and is the carotenoid associated with protection from prostate cancer. Lutein, another carotenoid in vegetables, accumulates in the eye and is associated with protection against the development of macular degeneration associated with aging. Given this range of activities from different carotenoids, it is important that your child receives all of these important phytonutrients, not just beta-carotene.

VITAMIN C

Clinical studies with vitamin C have suggested its use in counteracting or as a protective agent against many other conditions, such as colds and some infectious diseases. In addition to its protective effects against disease, vitamin C is necessary to support many normal processes in your body. Although many animals can make their own vitamin C, for humans, it is an essential vitamin, meaning that we cannot make it but must obtain it from the food we eat.

Vitamin C is the body's primary water soluble antioxidant, defending all aqueous areas of the body against free radicals that attack and damage normal cells. Free radicals have been shown to promote artery plaque build-up of atherosclerosis and diabetic heart disease, cause airway spasm that leads to asthma attacks, damage the cells of the colon so they become colon cancer cells, and contribute to the joint pain and disability seen in osteoarthritis and rheumatoid arthritis. This would explain why diets rich in vitamin C have been shown to be useful for preventing or reducing the severity of all of these conditions. In addition, vitamin C is vital for the proper functioning of the immune system, making it a nutrient to turn to for the prevention of recurrent ear infections, colds, and flu.

Feeding on vitamin C rich foods can be your child's cornerstone for strengthening the immune system. More in-depth studies have focused on vitamin C as one of the key nutrients that provide a vast range of protective activities. A higher body level of vitamin C is associated with a lower risk of strokes, atherosclerosis, and of dying from cardiovascular disease (CVD). Vitamin C may offer protection from CVD by its effect on cholesterol. Higher vitamin C levels in the body have been correlated with lower total cholesterol and LDL (harmful) cholesterol levels. Vitamin C also works together with vitamin E by restoring it to its functional, active form after it has been dismantled by free radicals.

Another recognized agent in the immune system is the interferons. These are proteins with antiviral activity, which are produced by cells infected by a virus and possibly also by malignant cells. Spreading to neighbouring cells, the interferons change them in such a way as to enable them to resist infection. There is some evidence that interferons help in the effort by the human body to control a developing cold or other infection or cancer. Different kinds of interferon are synthesized by different animal species. Human beings make about twenty different kinds of interferon molecules, with somewhat different activities, in different cells in the body. Interferon has attracted lively interest because very few drugs have any effectiveness against viral infections and cancer.

The suggestion that an increased intake of vitamin C would lead to the production of larger amounts of the interferons has been verified. Until more evidence becomes available about the value of injections of human interferon, it will be wise to follow the advice: "Take more vitamin C and make your own interferon!"

FROM THE LABS

A wound is an injury to the body caused by physical means, with disruption of the normal continuity of body structure. Accidents and surgical operations cause wounds. Broken bones are wounds. Since the healing of wounds requires the generation and laying down of collagen at the site, it would seem wise to call upon vitamin C in its role in the synthesis of collagen.

In an in-depth study conducted by Murad and his co-workers (1981-National Academy of Sciences, USA), an eight-fold increase in collagen production in tissue cultures supplied with vitamin C was demonstrated and their paper concluded with this observation: 'The clinical implications of this study are appreciable. The importance of ascorbate in wound healing has been recognized for years. Ascorbate is concentrated in wounded tissues and rapidly utilized during wound healing. Tensile strength of wounds and incidence of wound dehiscence are related to ascorbate levels. Because humans are dependent on dietary sources for ascorbate, deficiency is common in children, the elderly as well as sick and debilitated persons, who most commonly undergo surgical treatment. Such people may need supplemental ascorbate for optimal wound healing.'

The investigators pointed out that their results have high statistical significance in showing the acceleration of healing of pressure sores with 1 g per day of vitamin C. A larger intake should be even more effective. More than 30 years ago, it was reported that vitamin C and other vitamins in large doses have much value in the treatment of burns. (Brown, Farmer, and Franks, 1948;

Klasson, 1951; Yandell, 1951). It is, of course, reasonable that vitamin C should help in this healing process because it is required for the synthesis of collagen, which is a principal component of scar tissue, and of skin.

GETTING IT RIGHT

Vitamin C can easily be destroyed by prolonged storage and/or excess light. This is one of the reasons whole, fresh fruits and vegetables are a better source for this important nutrient than processed foods. Another reason whole foods are a better way of getting vitamin C is that it functions as a part of a nutrient team that includes such nutrients as vitamin E and the carotenoids, which are also in natural foods. The same compounds are often either not present or present in greatly reduced amounts in a processed food. Excellent sources of vitamin C including raw vegetables such as bell and chili peppers, broccoli, lettuce and fresh fruits such as kiwis, mangoes, apples, and oranges must be eaten mixed in specific combinations to extract all the benefits.

VITAMIN E

It is another essential vitamin found in natural foods that has significant health promoting advantages. An excellent antioxidant, it is important for the integrity of all of your cells' membranes – the protective gateways that allow nutrients in and wastes out, while keeping potentially destructive molecules from entering your cells. Vitamin E has been shown to protect from arterial damage, which it does by directly inhibiting the production of the damaging molecule, oxidized LDL cholesterol.

The importance of vitamin E can be seen from the fact that it helps to regenerate cells and preserve the lipid constituent of their membranes. In addition, a deficiency of vitamin E has been linked to neurological conditions and a higher risk of many types of cancers. There is no age which can be considered good to start on these compounds. The earlier you begin to supplement the diet in foods containing high amounts of these super foods, the more you gain. As the years pass, your children's body will give tangible proof of the effects these foods will be having.... retained youthful looks, lustrous hair, explosive energy and mental calmness which only perfect health can bring.

SELENIUM

Selenium, a mineral whose fundamental role is now recognized in all anti-free radicals mechanisms. It is integral to your health, wellbeing and rejuvenation. Like many minerals, selenium is used by a variety of different proteins in your body, like the enzymes that protect you from toxins and infectious bacteria. One especially important example is glutathione peroxidase, an enzyme that is present in most of your cells and is important in maintaining the level of glutathione, an antioxidant your body creates that protects your cells against damaging toxins and oxidants.

NONE OF THE BAD STUFF

The synergy of beneficial compounds inherent in completely natural foods may only be one piece of the puzzle as to why these foods are better for your children than un-whole foods. The other important aspect, complementing what natural foods do contain, is what whole foods do not contain.

Whole foods, by their nature, differ from refined foods in that they are not processed with an array of chemical additives. Some of these additives, although featured on the government's GRAS (generally recognized as safe) list and legally allowed to be added to the foods sold , are thought to compromise the body's structure and function, and are suggested to be related to a host of skin, pulmonary, and psycho-behavioural conditions.

The beauty of natural foods and their associated health benefits, seem to be a reflection of the natural synergy of all of their components: The totality of what they provide. And the MASTER KEY to their usage is a synergistic technique rather than mixing and matching haphazardly. Health promoting foods work better when consumed containing as much of their original complement of nutrients as possible. Studies exploring the relationship between diet and health consistently show health benefits from eating minimally processed whole foods; whereas, studies focusing solely on isolated compounds have yielded mixed or negative results.

SUPPORTING THE IMMUNE SYSTEM

Light, air, heat, time ... weaken all the above nutrients and lead to their degradation. To reap the full benefits, it is best to consume your food, the freshest possible. At the time of peeling fruits and vegetables or preparing them, keep them away from light and heat as much as possible

In general, to preserve your child's health and maximizing on the detailed plan as given ahead, it is necessary to eat everything in moderation, by remaining vigilant on their intake of zero nutrition and avoiding processed foods in favour of simple and natural dishes.

Healthy eating contributes to overall healthy growth and development, including healthy bones, skin, and energy levels; and a lowered risk of dental caries, eating disorders, constipation, malnutrition, and iron deficiency anaemia. The benefits of having a healthy, internally cleansed body with efficient functioning of all organs is a boon which can hardly be described but only experienced. You do not want your children to have any other type.

5 3 PANDIT PRINCIPLES

RESTRICTIVE DIET FOR KIDS MAY BACKFIRE

Parents who try to battle childhood junk eating epidemic by forbidding their kids to eat certain foods are not going to keep them healthy and may actually be making the situation worse. Parents need to play the critical role of guide cum friend in helping children make food choices that will allow them to maintain optimal health. However, success depends on using the right approach.

Parental attempts to help children with lower self-control by restricting their access to favourite snack foods can make the forbidden foods more attractive, thereby exacerbating the problem. A better idea for parents is to prepare similar dishes at home with nutrient dense ingredients, and when going out to eat help them learn some control by allowing them to choose between healthy options. And it is better to not keep restricted foods in the house. That way it is not necessary to constantly tell children they cannot have harmful foods.

FLETCHERIZE THE FOOD

Eating does not mean just swallowing the food as most children tend to do. Mastication in the mouth represents the first stage of digestion. It helps to grind food, to soak up saliva and degrade the fibre through the work of teeth; work of the stomach is thus facilitated. A famous quote, 'Nature will castigate those who don't masticate' is well known to health food advocates.

Children need to take time to look at what they are eating when food is served. At the sight, smell and flavour of food consumed, the brain sends nerve impulses to the stomach that secretes digestive enzymes needed to break down food. So, show them how to appreciate their food and take time to chew their food to ensure proper digestion, absorption and assimilation. You will also prevent bloating, stomach pain and heartburn.

EAT IN AN ORDERLY MANNER

Encourage everyone in the family, including children, to treat food with love and care. Eat only when sitting and encourage children to be calm during meals and not to eat while standing, walking, running, or playing, or while involved in other activities such as watching television. A meal eaten quickly does not leave the impression of having eaten. Indeed, the body needs time to develop satiety. The first signs appear about 20 minutes after the start of a meal; the brain detects the increase of sugar in the blood and then triggers the sensation of fullness. A good meal usually provides a pleasant feeling of satiety, that is to say a state of non-hunger.

Everyone may eat regularly two to three times per day, as much as they want, provided each meal includes the correct proportions of food and each mouthful is chewed thoroughly. Children may eat more frequently when necessary and may enjoy natural snacks from time to time, but again, try to discourage overeating. Habitual snacks can interfere with the eating of more regular and nutritionally complete meals.

A last word... Each child has different needs and wants. If you are sensitive to these differences, you can avoid many problems or sickness. Make suggestions to your children about what to eat if they are older and able to understand the importance of food. Point out how the foods they eat affect their behaviour. Explain how certain foods cause problems and how other foods are good for their health. However, for children to develop properly, you need to be flexible. Give them time to think about these ideas, and let them make the association between the foods they eat, and their physical and emotional health. Rather than imposing rules or using discipline to control their eating habits, let your children experience and discover things for themselves. If parents do not clearly understand the relationship between food and health, their method of handling these matters may become rigid or conceptual!

6 PLAY OR PERISH

Playing outside in all seasons is very important for a child's physical and mental health and wellbeing. Children who spend a great deal of time outdoors are usually happier, and eat and sleep better than children who spend much time indoors. Children need open spaces in which to run, jump, play, and enjoy freedom with little adult interference. You can, of course, accompany your children on outings to look after their safety. You can also join in the play when your children request it, or to help them get started. It is much easier for children to play outside if their homes are large. For children who live in apartments, parents may have to devote a little more time with them at the park or playground. It is helpful for children's social development if they can go to a park or playground every day to play with other children.

It is important to take your children to a variety of places such as the beach, zoo, park, farm, and the forest, instead of visiting the same place day after day. Taking children to many different places will stimulate their creativity, imagination, and desire to learn. They will have the opportunity to observe many types of people and social situations.

Developing physical strength is very important for a child's health and confidence. Encourage children to participate in as many sports and game activities as possible. Children who are physically strong are often happier, healthier, and more confident. If a child is physically weak, encouraging him to participate in sporting activities can help him overcome this problem.

BALANCING PLAY AND STUDY

While planning a young child's day, allow time for active play and for more quiet activities, such as looking at picture books, drawing, or studying. Parents can set aside time each day for toddlers to learn how to make things, or to read, or study together. If children develop these habits when they are young, they will usually continue them into adulthood. When children start school, it is important that they have time to sit quietly and read or do their homework. School children need a clean, quiet, and orderly space for studying and doing homework. It is better for them to finish their homework before watching television. If they stay up late watching television promising to do their homework afterward, they may become too tired to do it.

If children are not interested in studying, or in doing homework, or are not able to concentrate for long then dietary changes can usually help them by boosting brain power. *(Refer to **Superfoods-Make your child a genius**).*

A NEW LOOK AT EXERCISE

The main purpose of exercise is to increase circulation and intake of oxygen. This can be achieved by simple movements of the spine and various parts of the body with deep breathing.

WHAT HAPPENS IN MODERATE EXERCISE AND WHAT ROLE CAN IT PLAY IN MAKING YOUR CHILD'S IMMUNITY STRONGER?

A series of events occur which result in a greater flow of blood carrying an increased supply of oxygen and fuel to the active muscles. As muscle activity increases, muscle metabolism does likewise. Increased metabolism means greater heat production. The warming of muscles lowers their viscosity and increases the efficiency of work they perform.

In turn, the respiratory center responds with an increase in the frequency of impulses it rhythmically discharges. The greater number of impulses reaching the diaphragm and intercostal muscles induce stronger than usual contractions. Thus, breathing becomes deeper.

Faster and deeper breathing ventilates the lungs more thoroughly. A greater amount of carbon dioxide is removed in the expired air, **which prevents its concentration from rising too high in the blood, because too much carbon dioxide can increase the acidity of blood to a dangerous level.**

You can, knowing that it is largely a matter of training, increase your child's efficiency for strenuous tasks. Moderate and consistent exercises, besides making her feel better and relaxed, can help her body to become more adequate for the demands placed upon it. Moreover, a well trained body helps a great deal to train the mind and in turn be successful in life.

EXERCISE AND ARTERIES

The following is an extract from a medical journal: The chief killer of modern society is a disease known as arteriosclerosis or hardening of the arteries. The arteries become stiffened; their inner walls are lined with a coating of calcium. Sometimes they clog and crack, and the person dies of a stroke. Or they overwork the heart by trying to force blood through tubes narrowed due to calcium deposits and cause heart failure."

FROM THE LABS

Starling's LAW OF THE HEART: During exercise, more blood is returned to the heart than during rest. This is due to an increased venous return, which the contracting skeletal muscles introduce into the flow of blood. The pressure on the vessels by the contracting muscles pushes the blood along and the venous valves prevent the backward flow. Blood must move on towards the heart when pushed by the active muscles; as a result, the heart is better filled, which in turn stretches the fibres. When the fibres are stretched, they contract more forcibly, which means a stronger heartbeat and more blood being pumped out. The more forceful contraction, owing to the stretching of the muscles was discovered by the physiologist Starling and hence named.

Exercising can help to increase circulation and keep arteries elastic. Elasticity of muscles plays an important role in keeping the body youthful for years to come. Abnormal accumulation of fat, which is evenly or unevenly distributed in the muscular system due to inactivity, results in the hardening of body's muscular tissues. Exercise assists in removing this stiffness and prevents hardening.

EXERCISE AND JOINTS

If we study animals like dogs and cats, we notice that they often stretch and contract their spines after awakening. Infants move their spines naturally in a variety of positions. Flexibility of the spine is lost as the body grows. The average teenager can no longer touch the floor with his fingertips when his knees are straight. This type of ligamentous stiffening can be kept at a minimum through dynamized exercises and the body will be as pliable as a child's even at the age of eighty.

If posture and balance are good, ligaments have a long and elastic life. If not, they cause discomfort, pain, and trouble. Hence, it is essential that any form of exercise performed by children lays emphasis on the nature, function, and mobility of the spine and its ligaments.

As children grow older, their backbone stiffens because the ligaments become tighter. It must be remembered here that the ligamentous structures are continuous and if mobility is restricted in any area, the entire attachment is affected; this brings about general immobility of the body.

A new age style of yoga called power yoga pays great attention to the spinal column and other joints. Its dynamized exercises maintain an even supply of blood to every part of the body. Without a proper blood supply, the different tissues cannot be kept in good condition. For example, the application of a tight bandage interferes with the circulation of blood, lowers the temperature of the part that is poorly supplied, and causes a swelling. In normal cases, severe symptoms like swelling may not appear, but the various tissues cannot be kept in a healthy condition and efficiency to carry out various activities allotted to them diminishes without proper circulation. For a lasting effect and a permanent stretching of these ligaments, correct head and upper spine balance and flexibility are necessary, all of which can be accomplished by the daily practice of this form of yoga.

You will thus prevent a scenario in which your child's flexibility of the spine lessens at thirty and continues to decline at forty until at sixty and over, any bending may be difficult and painful. Starting at an early age will give an advantage over someone whose stiffened ligaments will not stretch at all and the body is held at the base of the skull, throughout the spine, pelvis, and knees by ligaments that have lost their elasticity.

EXERCISE AND ENDOCRINE GLANDS

What the Indian yogis knew long before, now the scientific community is advocating for the health of the endocrine glands. There are specific exercises that when practiced will have a regulating effect on your glandular system which in turn influences the emotions of the mind.

The endocrine glands include pancreas, thyroid, parathyroid, suprarenal, pituitary and the gonads.

Full growth, differentiation, and function of various parts of the body are possible only when there is a balanced activity of the internal secretions of the glands. Their secretions called hormones have an 'excite' or 'arouse' effect and these can be either immediate or delayed. They are relatively simple chemical substances, which must be either oxidized, or excreted after they have exerted their specific effects. If these secretions suffer, pathologic conditions in different parts of the body are rapidly established.

Thyroid is one of the most powerful agencies set up by nature to protect the body against toxins. When the thyroid hormone supply is inadequate for normal health, the rate of oxygen is reduced and the basal metabolism may be found as much as 40 per cent below normal for a person's age, height and weight. An abnormally low basal metabolism may produce certain kinds of obesity, which can be prevented by the practice of thyroid exercises.

Exercises from power yoga aim to restore the internal secretions of these glands to their normal levels with its dynamic poses. Different exercises can be done for strengthening respective glands. The entire endocrine system can be rejuvenated by exercising for a minimum 45 – 60 minutes a day.

EXERCISE AND CELLS

Exercising produces a salubrious effect on the minute cells of which the body is composed. The physical body is built of trillions of cells; each cell contains miniature life and energy for a definite function. Individual lives are really only bits of some degree of intelligence enabling the cells to work properly.

It is indispensible to know here that the cells of the body, which are used like building bricks, obtain their energy and nourishment through the blood stream. Without proper material, these cells cannot carry out their work. Children who are undernourished have not nearly the normal amount of blood cells and are consequently unable to have their system function optimally. The cells must have body-building material; there is only one way in which they can get this, and that is by means of nourishment from the food brought by the blood circulation, which is kept up easily through power yoga, or any simple yet gentle form of consistently done exercise.

EXERCISE AND DETOXIFICATION

Toxic matter and metabolic waste is eliminated from the body periodically. Anytime these poisons are allowed to accumulate, it will lead to disease and discomfort. Our lymphatic circulation, which is 'the sewer' for the cells in which they release their waste, moves only when we exercise. It is during contraction and expansion of the muscles that our lymph moves. While exercising, the toxicity is channeled to one of the eliminative organs and removed from the body. Doing some form of activity, which would move the muscles and work the joints is the minimum requirement for being fit, healthy, and having an incredibly strong immune system.

WHAT ARE DYNAMIZED EXERCISES?

These include power yoga, dancing, swimming or brisk walking with weights. They are high powered and spirited forms of exercises, which are made more dynamic from the usual style. Power yoga itself is a general term used to describe a fitness based approach to yoga. It puts emphasis on strength and flexibility. The advent of power yoga heralded yoga's current popularity in the western world, as people began to see yoga as a way to work out. It's all about working hard sensitively. It's about feeling good and looking good. Known for changing the face of how yoga is practiced in America, power yoga has quickly become one of the most widely known and respected educational method and yoga practice style to achieve personal transformation. It is truly a yoga practice without boundaries, and a personal development system that opens one up to a life of new possibilities.

Exercise forms like swimming, dancing, or brisk walking with weights can also be called dynamic when they are done vigorously and without rest. Swimming a certain number of laps in a fixed period can be considered dynamized and walking 4-5 kilometres with weights tied to your wrists and ankles, or stretching your limbs with simultaneous abdominal breathing is equivalent to dynamized exercise. All of these are safe methods of activities which can be done anywhere and do not require any specialized equipment or environment.

DYNAMIZED EXERCISES – A PANACEA

1. Increases strength and efficiency of the heart.
2. Lowers cholesterol.
3. Increases energy levels and stamina.
4. Increases bone mass – lowers risk of osteoporosis at a later age.
5. Helps to lose weight.
6. Will prevent hypertension and aids in stabilizing juvenile diabetes.
7. Promotes better sleep.
8. Moves food through the stream more quickly. Aids digestion.
9. Increases immunity to colds and coughs—more oxygen intake will flush the lungs.
10. Promotes a healthy back.
11. Relieves stress and anxiety.
12. Improves skin condition, blood circulation, lung's capacity.
13. Reduces headache.
14. Stimulates the lymphatic system.
15. Lifts one up mentally and emotionally.

There is no reason for not doing it. And consistency is the KEY.

INTERESTING!!

Unlike a pump to push the blood throughout the body that is, the heart, there is no organ to circulate waste matter out of the body. It is only exercising which moves this waste in the lymphatic circulation and out of your system.

7 SIGNS OF PERFECT HEALTH

1. BOUNDLESS ENERGY, CREATIVITY AND ENTHUSIASM

Healthy children play from morning to evening without growing bored or exhausted. Little ones may, of course, require a nap from time to time, but when they are awake, they are active and full of energy; so much so, in fact, that parents often have trouble keeping up with them. A good way to evaluate our own health is to consider how well we keep pace with our children.

A healthy child will approach life with a spirit of adventure. The energetic pursuit of dreams and ambitions including the capability to play, make believe, fantasize and daydream is a sign of good health and sound development. These capacities foster children's development, and help them realize their dreams throughout life.

2. A GOOD APPETITE

Children normally have healthy appetites, and not simply for food. Too much rich food or too many luxuries can spoil a child's appetite. For example, children are naturally attracted to sweet-to-taste foods. If they indulge in sugary snacks, sodas, candy, ice cream, or other poor quality foods, however, they will spoil their health. It is important for parents to use their better judgement when selecting their children's snacks and sweets.

A good appetite includes the desire for love, friendship, adventure, knowledge, and new experiences. Children are born with unlimited curiosity. This is reflected, as they grow, by their love of riddles, games, puzzles, and things that need to be figured out. They are always asking questions, and have a tremendous desire to participate in life. Children also seek love and friendship. They have no trouble making friends with children of their own age, with adults, or even with younger children or babies. Through their rich imaginations, they can also become friends with toys, animals, trees, rocks and almost anything they come in contact with. The ability to make friends is a sign that a child is healthy and well adjusted.

At the same time, children need opportunities to solve problems and confront challenges. This helps them to develop endurance, vitality, and patience. They will then be better equipped to deal with the challenges that arise during their lives. It is an expression of parental love to encourage moderation. When your children are old enough, explain to them that overindulgence can lead to dullness, stagnation, and weakness. Help them to understand that moderation actually strengthens and enhances their ability to participate in life. Moderation is not punishment, it is a means to further one's growth and development.

3. DEEP, SOUND SLEEP

When children are healthy, they enjoy good, sound sleep. Energetic physical and mental activity produces deep and restful sleep. When a healthy child sleeps, he is not bothered by nightmares or disturbing dreams. These come from imbalances in the brain and nervous system that result from excesses in the daily diet and environment. Television, movies, and other types of mental stimulation can also interact with a poor quality diet to produce disturbing and frightening dreams.

4. GOOD MEMORY AND IMAGINATION

Good memory is a sign of health. Memory provides the basis for all learning. Learning to walk, to control bowel movements and urination, and to speak, read, write, and do arithmetic all rest on the foundation of memory. Children learn to remember letters, numbers, and words, and to recreate scenery, people, and events, as well as emotions and feelings. Imagination, creativity, ambition, and future plans, or dreams are all based on memory. Memory is the foundation of health and happiness.

The ease with which children make friends is a result of their universal memory. Children intuitively remember their origin in the infinite universe, and realize instinctively that all people and things share the same origin. More relative or artificial distinctions such as race, occupation, nationality, or religious belief are usually not important to children and do not interfere with the desire to make friends. Children are naturally citizens of the world.

5. FREEDOM FROM ANGER, FEAR, AND OTHER NEGATIVE EMOTIONS

Negative emotions correlate to physical disorders. In Oriental countries, for example, anger is described as 'pain in the liver'. According to them, stagnation and other liver troubles frequently result from eating from too many animal foods, baked or overly cooked dishes, and minerals salts. Foods such as these can interfere with the natural flow of Earth's energy up the right side of the body. In this case, energy becomes stagnant and accumulates in the liver. Then, like a volcano, this stagnated energy periodically explodes in an outburst that we call anger. Children who are naturally healthy do not have this stagnation and thus, rarely experience anger.

Fear is related to an imbalance in the kidneys, often as a result of the over intake of fluids, saturated fats, sugar, animal proteins, and mineral salts. The kidneys stabilize the flow of energy in the body by harmonizing the energy that flows up through the right and down the left side of the body. When this balancing function is disturbed, a person loses confidence and stability.

We agree that the tendency towards fear is reinforced when parents strike or punish children, or when children experience artificial or painful procedures such as injections, operations, X-rays and so on. Teachers or other adults can instill fear when they assume an overly authoritarian or disciplinarian posture. Fear of nuclear war and failure to measure up to expectations, as well as fear of the future in general, are becoming common among children today. Underlying imbalances in the diet promote fear rather than a positive confidence in the future based on the desire to meet and overcome these challenges.

Abnormal mental or emotional conditions relate directly to imbalances in diet or upbringing. These imbalances distort the normal patterns of energy flow through the major organs and the body as a whole. As a result, these disruptions can prevent more healthy, emotional and intellectual responses.

6. A JOYFUL RESPONSE TO THE ENVIRONMENT

Healthy children respond joyfully to the changing world around them. They are able to respond in an original and flexible way, without more set or predictable patterns of thought and behaviour.

Open mindedness is also a characteristic of healthy children. They can entertain new ideas and situations without prejudice or preconceived notions. Children are usually much more adaptable than adults, who generally tend to be more set in their ways. Children are also very resilient; they are able to spring back from illness, failure, or difficulty and resume their play and activities with rapid speed.

7. WONDER, MARVEL AND APPRECIATION

Children find wonder everywhere. They intuitively sense a oneness with all things, and are grateful for their lives as human beings on this Earth. Their appreciation is often expressed simply in their joy of living, or in simple expressions of love and tenderness towards parents, brothers and sisters and friends.

part 2
THE 12 WEEKS INCREDIBLE IMMUNITY PLAN

The food pattern presented here contains no compromises. It is intended for those who desire to reach a chosen goal of becoming fitter, healthier, and more energetic in the shortest possible time. No limits have been placed on quantities, for the reason that some children require more than others do in order to be well nourished. You will be determining how much of any food your child wants to eat. It is well understood that eating a proper quantity means eating to a comfort level. You will not be adding any other food to this pattern, which will only complicate and reduce the digestive process. The specific pattern has an overall synergistic effect on the body and each meal is to be fully digested, absorbed, and assimilated to extract maximum nutrients from it for regeneration and boosting the immune system.

WEEK ONE

MONDAY

Early morning: Emerge Regenerated
Breakfast: Boundless Energy
Lunch: Of choice with Raw Paw Salad
Evening: Blood Detox
Dinner: Of choice

TUESDAY

Early morning: Energy booster
Breakfast: Chinese Tossed Vegetables
Lunch: Of choice with The Blood Fixer
Evening: Taste bubble
Dinner: Of choice

WEDNESDAY

Early morning: Fuel for Beauty
Breakfast: Feast Today
Lunch: Of choice with Transformator
Evening: Sweet 'n' Magical
Dinner: Of choice

THURSDAY

Early morning: Let 'er' Rip
Breakfast: Celebrate Childhood
Lunch: Of choice with Natural Brain Protector
Evening: Children's Favourite
Dinner: Of choice

FRIDAY

Early morning: Emerge Regenerated
Breakfast: Robust Transition
Lunch: Of choice with Fresh 'n' Juicy
Evening: Blood Detox
Dinner: Of choice

SATURDAY

Early morning: Energy Booster
Breakfast: Tasty Tangles
Lunch: Of choice with Immune Power
Evening: Taste Bubble
Dinner: Of choice

SUNDAY

Early morning: Fuel for Beauty
Breakfast: Southern Delicacy
Lunch: Of choice with Energy Reviver
Evening: Sweet 'n' Magical
Dinner: Of choice

WEEK TWO

MONDAY

Early morning: Revitalizer
Breakfast: Colour of Health
Lunch: Of choice with Dream Salad
Evening: Immunity Raiser
Dinner: Of choice

TUESDAY

Early morning: Ride 'em' High
Breakfast: Brilliance Craft
Lunch: Of choice with Secret of Angels
Evening: Infuse your immunity
Dinner: Of choice

WEDNESDAY

Early morning: Veggie Magic
Breakfast: Walnutty Sandwiches
Lunch: Of choice with Knock Out
Evening: Sweet Blessings
Dinner: Of choice

THURSDAY

Early morning: Let 'er' Rip
Breakfast: Fortune for Vitals
Lunch: Of choice with London Special
Evening: Children's Favourite
Dinner: Of choice

FRIDAY

Early morning: Revitalizer
Breakfast: Turbo Charger
Lunch: Of choice with Perfect 10
Evening: Immunity Raiser
Dinner: Of choice

SATURDAY

Early morning: Ride 'em' High
Breakfast: Tempted
Lunch: Of choice with Parisian Salad
Evening: Infuse your immunity
Dinner: Of choice

SUNDAY

Early morning: Veggie Magic
Breakfast: Master your Metabolism
Lunch: Of choice with Whizz Bang
Evening: Sweet Blessings
Dinner: Of choice

WEEK THREE

MONDAY

Early morning: Emerge Regenerated
Breakfast: Morning Mantra
Lunch: Of choice with Booster
Evening: Blood detox
Dinner: Of choice

TUESDAY

Early morning: Energy Booster
Breakfast: Chinese Tossed Vegetables
Lunch: Of choice with Dream Salad
Evening: Taste bubble
Dinner: Of choice

WEDNESDAY

Early morning: Fuel for Beauty
Breakfast: Tasty Tangles
Lunch: Of choice with Secret of Angels
Evening: Sweet 'n' Magical
Dinner: Of choice

THURSDAY

Early morning: Let 'er' Rip
Breakfast: Boundless Energy
Lunch: Of choice with Perfect 10
Evening: Children's Favourite
Dinner: Of choice

FRIDAY

Early morning: Revitalizer
Breakfast: Turbo Charger
Lunch: Of choice with Transformator
Evening: Immunity Raiser
Dinner: Of choice

SATURDAY

Early morning: Ride 'em' High
Breakfast: Southern Delicacy
Lunch: Of choice with London Special
Evening: Infuse your immunity
Dinner: Of choice

SUNDAY

Early morning: Veggie Magic
Breakfast: Tempted
Lunch: Of choice with Energy Reviver
Evening: Sweet Blessings
Dinner: Of choice

After completing three weeks of **'the incredible immunity plan'**, repeat the cycle four times to complete 12 weeks. It takes a minimum of twelve weeks for the body to adapt to the new foods, absorb and assimilate the nutrients to a deep tissue level.

After the period of 12 weeks is over, you can continue to serve your children foods from the plan as per their liking and your convenience.

Another way to really benefit from this book will be to follow 'the incredible immunity plan' again after 6 months to renew and recharge the body and boost up the immune system. Thereafter you may use the plan once a year to support your children's growing needs and protect them from infections and illness.

NOT TO MISS SPECIAL POINTERS:

- You are advised to avoid white flour products and any food containing preservatives (food which is tinned, packed, packaged or tetra packed) in your child's diet during the period of 12 weeks when you are following it. The earlier chapters clearly illuminate how these elements that can not only delay, but prevent you from getting any results by weakening the immune system.
- **Ingredient not available:** There can be times in the year when you do not have a specific ingredient at hand. There is no reason to get stressed. You can substitute another recipe from the same section taking care not to repeat the same thing consecutively for a few days.

  It is easy to fall into a trap of making something you are used to or convenient to you. It is even easier to fall into a pattern where you end up making only those recipes which your child has liked.

  Do not go down this track. Some children can take more time to adapt to different tastes than the ones they are used to, but all of them finally change. From experience we know that sometimes a food has to be served nearly 19-20 times before it becomes accepted as a loved recipe.

- **Child feels hungry in the evening:** We are aware that the snacks we have given in the evening for children are light on the stomach. Yet these are highly potent mixtures made from nutritionally dense foods and act when they are given without any accompaniment. Please avoid serving something at this time to 'top up the stomach' after they have partaken the snacks as prescribed.

- **What about milk?** The entire 12 weeks plan takes into account the calcium intake for your child during this period. We have carefully incorporated different sources of calcium like nuts, soymilk, tofu, yoghurt, grains and greens and many more. These sources have far more 'bioavailable calcium' than milk. Please note milk is not the only and not the least 'best source' of calcium for children. In fact, after following this food pattern most of the children under our care increased in height and became taller without drinking milk every day.

  You can always return to milk after the 12 weeks are over. We are certain you will thank us for the break.

part 3
FOOD FOR LIFE

Let's take a voyage through different elements of food which are nutritionally dense and thereby are important to be included in the diet plan of every child.

NATURE'S BOUNTY–FRUITS

APPLES

WHAT MAKES A TRULY TASTY APPLE?

Apples have a moderately sweet, refreshing flavour and a tartness that is present to a greater or lesser degree depending on the variety. The flavour is a magical blend of tartness, sweetness, bitterness, and aroma that awakens the senses. The sweetness, 9 per cent to 12 per cent of the fruit, comes from sucrose and fructose, two forms of natural sugar. The acid content consists of 90 per cent malic acid and 10 per cent citric acid. The malic acid content can make up 0.4 per cent to 1 per cent of the fruit. The familiar aroma is a mysterious blend of 250 trace chemicals contained in the fruit, such as volatile esters, alcohols, and aldehydes.

AN APPLE A DAY

Apples are such commonly consumed fruits that it's easy to overlook their amazing and unique health benefits. Apples combine certain nutrients in a way that sets them apart from all other fruits and makes them a food of choice for achieving several health goals. Here's what apples can do for you when it comes to your health:

Easy on the digestion, acids in the apple inhibit fermentation in the intestines. Their high fiber content adds bulk aiding the digestive process, making elimination natural and comfortable. Apples contain pectin, a soluble fiber which encourages growth of beneficial bacteria in the digestive tract.

Green apples act as a liver and gall bladder cleanser and may aid in softening gall stones. Because of their high water content, apples are cooling and moistening and aid in reducing fever. Apples sweetened with honey are beneficial for a dry cough and may help remove mucous from the lungs.

Today, medical practitioners are beginning to recognize that the apple's abundant quantity of pectin is an aid in reducing high cholesterol as well as blood sugar, a wonder food for people with coronary artery disease and diabetes.

You'll get impressive amounts of flavonoids in the skins and pulp of apples, and these flavonoids have plenty of tricks up their sleeve for helping protect your heart's health. Many flavonoids provide antioxidant protection; some help prevent excessive and unwanted inflammation; others help prevent too much clumping together of blood platelets; and still others help regulate blood pressure and overproduction of fat in your liver cells. Flavonoids have also shown to improve problems with heart disease once it has occurred.

ANTI-ASTHMA AND LUNG SUPPORT

Apples have stood out amongst other fruits when it comes to general support of lung function and lung health. Flavonoids unique to apple including phloridzin, are thought to play a potentially key role in the special ability of apples to support lung health.

Interesting!!

Apple is actually a member of the rose family.

APRICOTS

That such a wonderful food can also be good for your health is one of life's little bonuses! The Hunza people are renowned for living healthily into their nineties or longer and the population has a negligible cancer rate. Part of their mineral rich diet is their apricots that are allowed to dry on the tree, taking on a crinklier and browner appearance than we are used to seeing.

FROM THE LABS

Apricots contain phytochemicals called carotenoids, which contain the powerful antioxidant, lycopene. The health facts for these delectable fruit are:

1. Apricots provide fibre to assist in healthy digestion and digestive function.
2. Apricots contain high levels of potassium which help maintain an adequate blood pressure.
3. Apricots are high in beta-carotene, an antioxidant with significant health promoting properties such as fighting cancer cells and lowering the risk from heart disease, keeping the central nervous system healthy, and maintaining your vision for years.

With every bite of apricots you are helping your body fight infection, repair damaged tissues, build strong teeth and bones, and all this with a fruit that is naturally fat and cholesterol-free, and a good source of dietary fibre and potassium.

> ### Interesting!!
>
> *According to Greek mythology experts, the 'golden apples' of Hesperides were actually apricots. They were the fruit Hercules was ordered to pick for his eleventh task.*

BANANAS

They are surely the best known tropical fruit, and one of the most healthy and versatile. Neatly packaged in their attractive easy-peel skins, hygienically enclosing the sweet, creamy-white, floury flesh, bananas are the perfect convenience food.

FROM THE LABS

Because of their impressive potassium content, bananas are highly recommended by doctors for patients whose potassium is low. One large banana, about 9 inches in length, packs 602 mg of potassium. That same large banana has 2 grams of protein and 4 grams of fibre. No wonder the banana was considered an important food to boost the health of malnourished children.

Researchers have also found that 2 or 3 bananas a day are beneficial in treating children with coeliac disease, an intolerance to grains that contain gluten such as wheat, rye, oats, and barley.

Vitamins and minerals are abundant in the banana, offering 123 I.U. of vitamin A for the large size. A full range of B vitamins are present with 0.07 mg of Thiamine, 0.15 mg of riboflavin, 0.82 mg niacin, 0.88 mg vitamin B6 and 29 mcg of folic acid. There are even 13.8 mg of vitamin C.

On the mineral scale, calcium counts in at 9.2 mg, magnesium 44.1 mg, with trace amounts of iron and zinc. Putting all the nutritional figures together clearly shows that the banana is among the healthiest of fruits.

> ### Interesting!!
>
> *In his campaign in India in 327 BCE, Alexander the Great relished his first taste of the banana, an usual fruit he saw growing on tall trees. He is even credited with bringing the banana from India to the western world.*

DATES

Dates are termed as the crown of sweets and an ideal food, easily digested. It gives extra energy to a tired human body within half an hour after taking it. It is said that 'taking one date in a day will help you to maintain your healthy eyes for your lifetime'. They are quiet effective in guarding against night blindness. Dates are considered to be the best diet for women expecting a baby. They nourish the foetus and the mother-to-be.

Uncountable health benefits. This fruit is affluent in natural fibre and contains oil, calcium, sulphur, iron, potassium, phosphorus, manganese, copper and magnesium which are advantageous for health. It is said that one date is the minimum requirement of a balanced and healthy diet. It helps in fighting constipation, intestinal disorders, weight gain, heart problems, sexual weakness, diarrhoea and abdominal cancer. Their nutrients have dates—the best nourishment for muscles development.

Date is termed to be a laxative food, thus it is beneficial for people suffering from constipation.

The nicotinic content present in them is said to be beneficial for curing any kinds of intestinal disorders. Continuous intake of this delicious fruit helps to maintain a check on the growth of the pathological organisms, and helps in the rise of friendly bacteria in the intestines.

They work as a powerful tonic for all age groups. They work better than any medicine, or body building supplement since they are natural, and do not bear any side effects in the body.

ENERGIZERS

A serving of power-packed dates contains 31 grams of carbohydrates, makes them a power house of energy. Carbohydrates include 3 grams of dietary fibre and 29 grams of naturally occurring sugars such as fructose, glucose and sucrose to provide quick energy, readily used by the body. Dates are a perfect energy boosting snack.

Ounce per ounce, pound for pound, dates are one of the best natural sources of potassium. Potassium is an essential mineral your body needs to maintain muscle contractions including the vital heart muscle. Potassium is needed to maintain a healthy nervous system and to balance the body's metabolism. Dates contain a variety of B complex vitamins – thiamine, riboflavin, niacin, vitamin B6 and antithetic acid. These vitamins have a variety of functions in maintaining a healthy body; to metabolize carbohydrates and maintain blood glucose levels, fatty acids for energy, and help make haemoglobin, the red and white blood cells.

Interesting!!

The date palm was important to three of the world's major religious groups; the Jews, the Muslims and the Christians.

FIGS

The fig tree is a symbol of abundance, of fertility, of sweetness. These oval or pear shaped fruits are among the most luscious of all and can be eaten fresh or dried.

Figs feature a complex texture that combines the chewiness of their flesh, the smoothness of their skin, and the crunchiness of their seeds. Since fresh figs are so delicate and perishable, some of their mystique comes from their relative rarity. Because of this, majority of figs are dried, either by exposure to sunlight or through an artificial process, creating a sweet and nutritious dried fruit that can be enjoyed throughout the year.

FROM THE LABS

Figs are rich in calcium, iron, phosphorus and potassium. Vitamin C and the B group vitamins are also present in small quantities. They are also high in fibre. Figs have the highest overall mineral content of all common fruits. Figs are fat-free, sodium-free and cholesterol-free. One of their virtues is to assist the bowels in their normal peristaltic movements while their bone building ability makes them indispensable in any household.

KIWI

These cylindrical shaped fruits are covered with a light brown fuzzy skin, which looks very dull in comparison with the beautiful bright green interior, with its crown of tiny edible seeds arranged around a white core. The flavour is delicate, yet refreshing and tangy.

Kiwi fruits are rich in many vitamins, flavonoids and minerals. In particular, they contain a high amount of vitamin C (more than oranges), as much potassium as bananas and a good amount of beta-carotene.

Vitamin C is a water soluble antioxidant that has been proven to protect our body from free radicals. Vitamin E has been proven to have similar effects, but is fat soluble and thus is complimentary to vitamin C in its functions. Kiwi fruits contain both these vitamins in high amount, which help protect our body against free radicals from all fronts.

In tests done for the benefits of eating this fruit, shortness of breath was reduced by 32 per cent, night time cough by 27 per cent severe wheeze by 41 per cent, chronic cough by 25 per cent, and runny nose by 28 per cent. This results is not only traceable to the content in vitamin C or potassium, but in substances which are still largely unknown contained in kiwi fruit. These substances are most likely flavonoids that help protect our cells from oxidative damage, and are therefore considered very helpful in protecting our DNA from mutations and damage.

Interesting!!

A lady initiated the import of these fruits into the United States in 1962, but to meet what was felt to be burgeoning demand, changed its name from Chinese gooseberry to kiwi fruit, in honour of the native bird of New Zealand, the kiwi, whose brown fuzzy coat resembled the skin of this unique fruit.

MANGO

Revered not only for their exotic sweetness and juicy quality, mangoes are known for their many health blessings. They contain an enzyme similar to papain in papayas, a soothing digestive aid. These proteolytic enzymes that break down proteins are effective meat tenderizers regularly used in tropical countries where mangoes are grown. The enzyme list continues with magneferin, katechol oxidase, and lactase that not only protect the mango from insects, but help humans by stimulating metabolism and purifying the intestinal tract.

BASKET OF BENEFITS

In India, mangoes are used as blood builders. Because of their high iron content, they are suggested for treatment of anaemia and are beneficial to women during pregnancy and menstruation. People who suffer from muscle cramps, stress, and heart problems can benefit from the high potassium and magnesium content. These minerals also help those with acidosis.

A rather startling result has been obtained while testing mangoes in the laboratory. Mango juice was poured into a test tube that contained viruses. Shortly, the viruses were destroyed.

One medium mango is a mighty impressive, self-contained package of vitamins, minerals and antioxidants. Like most fruits, the mango is low in protein, about 1 gram for a medium size, but you can certainly benefit from its 3.7 grams of fibre.

Mango is a shining star in the beta-carotene realm, summing up at 8061 IU for that same medium size. If you're looking for a boost in potassium, look no further than a medium mango with its 322.92 mg. It's the perfect fruit to replenish energy after heavy physical exercise like jogging or working out. Magnesium content is 18.63 mg.

Although these figures will vary with the different varieties and different sizes, there is little doubt that the mango is an exceptional fruit, not only for its high ranking nutrients, but also for its intense, zesty and delightful flavour that just may taste like paradise itself.

Interesting!!

It is said that Buddha was given the gift of a whole grove of mango trees where he could rest whenever he wished. From that time on, the mango tree was held in awe as capable of granting wishes.

MELONS

Melons fall into two main categories – summer fruit and winter fruit. The summer varieties include melons with cross hatched skin that looks like a brown netting. Winter melons have a smooth or finely ridged pale, or bright yellow rind.

FROM THE LABS

The ideal summer fruit, melon's cooling ability is not so surprising when we realize its weight is 95 per cent water, while the sugar content is only 5 per cent. Melons are a health conscious person's delight! It's rich in natural sugar, has almost zero fat, and its flavour is positively ambrosial. One fourth of a medium sized melon provides 80 per cent of the RDA for both vitamins A and C.

The dark orange coloured melon – cantaloupe really shines when it contains vitamin A. One fourth of a medium cantaloupe provides a hearty 4450 IU. The same quarter of a cantaloupe also provides 2 per cent of the RDA for both iron and calcium, offers 1 gram of fibre and 1 gram of protein.

Melons of the variety cantaloupe, muskmelon, casaba, honeydew or crenshaw provides a moderate amount of B vitamins, folic acid along with minerals like potassium and calcium.

PROMOTES LUNG HEALTH – INCREASES YOUR STAMINA

Vitamin A precursor – beta-carotene in the deep orange melon strengthens the lungs, improving oxygen intake. There is a continuous, enhanced detoxification of blood which translates into better endurance in physical activity. If you or someone you love is a smoker, or if you are frequently exposed to secondhand smoke, then making a super food such as cantaloupe, part of your healthy way of eating can not only protect you from premature aging of the skin and capillaries, it may save your life at the same time.

Interesting!!

A Middle Eastern proverb states, 'He who fills his stomach with melons is like he who fills it with light—there is baraka (a blessing) in them'.

ORANGES

No family of fruits seems to store up sunshine more successfully than citrus fruits. Golden oranges and tangerines, yellow lemons and sweet limes – their glowing colours light up a room, and the wonderful scent of their essential oils tempts the taste buds.

From the labs: In recent research studies, the healing properties of oranges have been associated with a wide variety of phytonutrient compounds.

World Health Organization's recent draft report, "Diet, Nutrition and the Prevention of Chronic Disease," concludes that a diet that features orange fruits also offers protection against cardiovascular disease due to oranges' folate, which is necessary for lowering levels of the cardiovascular risk factor, homocysteine; their potassium, which helps lower blood pressure, protecting against stroke and cardiac arrhythmias; and the vitamin C, carotenoids and flavonoids found in them, all of which have been identified as having protective cardiovascular effects.

The CSIRO Report also includes evidence of positive effects associated with citrus consumption in studies for arthritis, asthma, Alzheimer's disease and cognitive impairment, Parkinson's disease, macular degeneration, diabetes, gall stones, multiple sclerosis, cholera, gingivitis, optimal lung function, cataracts, ulcerative colitis and Crohn's disease.

An orange has over 170 different phytonutrients and more than 60 flavonoids, many of which have been shown to have anti-inflammatory, anti-tumour, and blood clot inhibiting properties as well as strong antioxidant effects.

UNIQUE VITAMIN C ACTIVITY

Free radical damage to cellular structures and other molecules can result in painful inflammation, as the body tries to clear out the damaged parts. Vitamin C, which prevents free radical damage that triggers the inflammatory cascade, is thus associated with reduced severity of inflammatory conditions, such as asthma, osteoarthritis, and rheumatoid arthritis.

Free radicals also oxidize cholesterol. Only after being oxidized does cholesterol stick to the artery walls, building up in plaques that may eventually grow large enough to impede or fully block blood flow, or rupture to cause a heart attack or stroke. Since vitamin C can neutralize free radicals, it can help prevent the oxidation of cholesterol.

In oranges, vitamin C is part of a matrix involving many beneficial phytochemicals (for example, cyanidin-3-glucoside, flavanones and carotenoids). An increasing number of studies have shown a greater absorption of the nutrients in citrus when taken not as singly as supplements, but when consumed within the fruit in which they naturally appear along with all the other biologically active phytonutrients that citrus fruits contain.

In addition to oranges' phytonutrients, vitamin C and fibre, they are a good source of thiamine, folate, vitamin A (in the form of beta-carotene), potassium and calcium.

Interesting!!

Citrus fruits are protective against overweight and obesity. You do have to eat them separately from cooked food, or vegetable salads to get this effect.

PAPAYA

The humble papaya is a storehouse of vitamins and nutrients. Native to central America, it was introduced into India by the Dutch sometime in the sixteenth century. From here it spread to all the south Asian countries. A tropical fruit with a sweet taste, papaya was named 'the most nutritious fruit' by the Centre for Science, USA while years ago Christopher Columbus called it 'the fruit of the angels'.

Papaya is invaluable as a health tonic as it contains all the principal constituents of food. It is rich in vitamins A, C, B factors and also contains ample amounts of proteins, minerals like potassium and magnesium, fibre and carbohydrates. The sugar in the fruit is an energy provider.

As a source of beta-carotene which is a precursor of vitamin A, papaya is unrivalled by any other fruit except perhaps the mango. A small papaya has oodles of taste, little to no fat, one gram of fibre and nearly a day's worth of vitamin C and beta-carotene, as well as a fair amount of potassium and folic acid. Since papaya is relatively cheap, available in all seasons and in most places, it gives maximum nutritional returns for the money spent.

The fruit has been revered for its medicinal value since days of yore. Modern scientific investigations into the properties of the papaya have confirmed many of the ancient beliefs in its virtues. The most important of these virtues is the discovery of a protein digesting enzyme in the milky juice or latex, which is carried in a network of vessels throughout the plant. The enzyme is similar to pepsin in its digestive action and is reputed to be so powerful that it can digest 200 times its own weight in protein. Its effect is to assist the body's own enzymes in assimilating the maximum nutritional value from food to provide energy and body building materials. This enzyme called 'Papain' is found in the raw (green) papaya.

Papaya can work the numerous miracles in the body including:

RECHARGE YOUR DIGESTION

Papain in the raw papaya is highly beneficial in the deficiency of gastric juice, excess of unhealthy mucous in the stomach, in dyspepsia and intestinal irritation. The ripe fruit, if eaten regularly, corrects habitual constipation, bleeding piles and chronic diarrhoea. Evidence suggests that raising one's digestive enzyme levels can strengthen the immune system. The enzymes in papaya can also enhance carbohydrate and fat digestion.

SHIELD AGAINST BACTERIA

Other phytonutrients in green papaya help create a healthier intestinal tract by restoring proper intestinal flora. Carpaine, an alkaloid found in green papaya has antibacterial properties that neutralize many types of harmful bacteria and parasites.

The ripe fruit rids the body of constipation, bleeding piles and chronic diarrhoea. Regular consumption of papaya can help prevent night blindness, an ailment caused by vitamin A deficiency, which is common in many Indian children. Pieces of papaya laid on wounds and surgical incisions have been reported to speed up their healing. Beta-carotene, which is present in large quantities in papaya, is also an antioxidant and cancer preventer.

Interesting!!

According to legend, this modest fruit once saved the life of a British Major, whose thigh was bleeding profusely after a jeep accident. A passing doctor broke a papaya and pressed it to his wound, which arrested the bleeding. This inspired a movie 'The scent of the Green Papaya' that was nominated in 1994 for an Academy Award for the best foreign film.

PEAR

Pears are not only a juicy, sweet tasting treat, but they are also very nutritious, higher in fibre than apples, and easier to digest. Because they are so easy to digest and are hypoallergenic, pears are often introduced to babies as their first fruit. Pectin, which is the fibre found in Pears, helps to lower cholesterol, improve cardiovascular function and promote intestinal health.

Along with pectin, pears are a wonderful source of vitamin C and copper, which together, provide powerful antioxidant protection, helping to fight off disease and even some cancers by protecting the body from free radicals. These fruits are an excellent source of vitamin B2, vitamin E, folic acid and potassium.

> ### Interesting!!
> *A member of the rose family, the pear fruit's origin dates back to the Middle East. It is one of the world's oldest cultivated fruits.*

PINEAPPLE

Pineapples have exceptional juiciness and a vibrant tropical flavour that balances the tastes of sweet and tart. The area closer to the base of the fruit has more sugar content and therefore a sweeter taste and more tender texture.

ANTI-INFLAMMATORY CUM CLEANSER

Bromelain is a complex mixture of substances that can be extracted from the stem and fruit core of the pineapple. Excessive inflammation, excessive coagulation of blood, and certain types of tumour growths may all be reduced by the regular eating of this fruit. It is an excellent source of the trace mineral manganese, which is an essential co-factor in a number of enzymes important for energy production and antioxidant defenses.

The natural bromelain digests debris of mucous in the intestinal tract, cleaning it up and strengthening the system from further colds and flu's.

> ### Interesting!!
> *Since pineapples are very perishable, and modes of transportation to bring them stateside from the Caribbean Islands were relatively slow centuries ago, fresh pineapples were a rarity that became coveted by the early American colonists. While glazed, sugar-coated pineapples were a luxurious treat, it was the fresh pineapple itself that became the sought after true symbol of prestige and social class. In fact, the pineapple, because of its rarity and expense, was such a status item in those times that all a party hostess had to do was to display the fruit as part of a decorative centerpiece, and she would be awarded more than just a modicum of social awe and recognition.*

POMEGRANATE

The pomegranate is sweet, but the pomegranate is tart. The pomegranate is tough and wrinkled, but when cut open it glistens with ruby-like seeds.

FROM THE LABS

The pomegranate provides a substantial amount of potassium, is high in fibre, and contains vitamin C and niacin. Research conducted by Michael Aviram of the Lipid Research Laboratory at the Technion – Israel Institute of Technology has revealed the antioxidant properties of the fruit. Preliminary studies have indicated the juice of the fruit to possess almost three times the total antioxidant ability of green tea or red wine.

Interesting!!

Muhammad, the Prophet whose visions laid the foundation of Islam, considered the pomegranate to be a precious fruit filled with nutrition, bringing both emotional and physical peace.

PRUNES

Prunes are nutritious fruits that are extremely fun to eat since they have a sweet, deep taste and a sticky, chewy texture. Prunes are actually dried plums, more specifically the dried version of European plums, including the Agen variety.

GOOD DIGESTION IS EQUAL TO REMAINING FIT

Prunes are renowned as a mild, folk loric laxative, and ancient Egyptian and Greek physicians once prescribed prunes to patients with gastrointestinal problems. Because prunes are loaded with fibre and natural laxatives, they help in correcting and encouraging regular bowel movements. They promote better digestion. Not only do prunes help in producing good bacteria but the fibre collects unnecessary fat and helps move it through the colon. This helps with the bowel movements and keeps the colon free from backing up and causing pain.

Antioxidant rich food like prunes, are known to combat free radicals and prevent certain cancers and diseases, but the good news is antioxidants in prunes also keep the body fit and prevent vision loss.

The prune's nutritional composition combined with its sweetness makes it an excellent and tasty addition to your child's diet. Prunes are bursting with:

1. Phytochemicals
2. Natural Laxative Dihydrophenylisatin
3. Iron
4. Dietary Fiber
5. Potassium
6. Vitamins A, B3 and B6

> ### Interesting!!
>
> *Prunes were historically a French delicacy. Currently, in the new age they are relished as a means to reduce high blood pressure and preventing atherosclerosis.*

STONE FRUIT

It is a woody-skinned, smooth fruit 5-15 cm in diametre. The skin of some forms of the fruit is so hard, it must be cracked open with a hammer. It has numerous seeds, which are densely covered with fibrous hairs and are embedded in a thick, gluey, aromatic pulp. The fruit is eaten fresh or dried.

During 'the plan', this fruit will have a large role to play. The benefits you get are attributed to the tannin present in the fruit.

Bael fruit is good for digestion. It helps to destroy worms in the intestine and is a good remedy for digestive disorders. While the juice of the fruit is recommended for treating chronic dysentery, the laxative property of wood apple's pulp helps to avoid constipation. Bael fruit is used for healing people with peptic ulcer or piles. Bael leaves contain tannin, which reduces inflammation, and can be added to salads.

Eating the fruit or drinking the 'sherbet' made from it acts as a blood cleanser. Since Bael fruit is rich in vitamin C, it is anti-scorbutic and prevents scurvy. It contains natural sugar and a rich fragrant flavour giving a boost of energy to the body. Regular consumption of wood apple is advised for people with kidney complaints. As a good source of beta-carotene, a precursor of vitamin A, and significant quantities of the B vitamins thiamine and riboflavin, wood apples cure and correct liver problems and is often found as an ingredient in cardiac tonics.

> ### Interesting!!
>
> *This fruit is called elephant apple because it's the favourite of elephants. It gets the name wood apple because of its hard wooden shell.*

FASCINATING WORLD OF SPICES

BISHOP'S WEED

The trade name of this spice, ajwain is based on the Indian name which is derived from adarjawan. Ajwain or Bishop's weed has been used as a carminative medicine from the time of Charaka, Sushruta, and greek physicians like Dioscrides and Galen.

The seeds are stimulant and useful in counteracting spasmodic disorders. The oil of ajwain is an almost colourless to brownish liquid with a characteristic odour and a sharp hot taste.

FROM THE LABS

An analysis of ajwain seeds shows calcium, phosphorus, iron, carotene, thiamine, riboflavin and niacin amongst the vitamins and minerals in it.

The seeds are useful in the treatment of migraine and delirium. The oil present in them is beneficial in the treatment of rheumatic and neuralgic pains. They are useful in the treatment of common cold since they possess a remarkable power to open up clogged and congested nasal passages. They increase appetite, improve digestion and tone up the muscles of the digestive tract.

CARAWAY

It falls into both categories of herb and spice, as it is the seeds that are used primarily, but if you grow it on your own, the leaves and the root are also edible. Caraway has been found in food dating back to 3000 BC, making it one of the oldest cultivated spices.

The seeds, brown in colour, are hard and sharp to touch. They have a pleasant odour, aromatic flavour, somewhat sharp taste and leave a somewhat warm feeling in the mouth. Caraway seeds can hold their flavour for months stored in airtight containers and kept away from light.

FROM THE LABS

An analysis of caraway shows it to contain appreciable moisture, protein, fat, substantial amounts of carbohydrates besides ash, calcium, phosphorus, sodium, potassium, iron, thiamine, riboflavin and niacin. It also contains vitamins C and A.

The caraway seeds are considered useful in activating the glands, besides increasing the action of the kidneys. It is characterized as an excellent 'house cleaner' for the body. They are useful in strengthening the functions of stomach. They have carminative properties which means they help with gas and digestion.

CARDAMOM

It is best to buy the whole pods as ground cardamom quickly loses flavour. This 'queen of spices' was chewed by Moghul emperors of India as a breath freshener, a tradition that still exists today. The Arabs attributed many qualities to it (it features regularly in the Arabian Nights) and the ancient Indians regarded it as a cure for obesity.

This rich green spice has a pungent, warm, and aromatic bouquet with a flavour that's warm and eucalyptine with camphorous and lemony undertones.

A stimulant and carminative, cardamom forms a flavouring agent. It also forms the basis for medicinal preparations for indigestion and flatulence using other substances, entering into a synergetic relationship with them. It is a key digestive with anti-spasmodic properties.

Interesting!!

The ancient Egyptians chewed cardamom seeds as a tooth cleaner; the Greeks and Romans used it as a perfume and the Vikings came upon cardamom about one thousand years ago.

CHILLI

Aside from their eye-opening flavour, perhaps the most surprising feature of chilli peppers is their vitamin C content: 91 milligrams in one-fourth cup of fresh chilies. Though we don't eat chilli peppers in large quantities, the amount of vitamin C is still significant. Red chillies are full of beta-carotene.

FROM THE LABS

Most interesting to researchers today, however, is capsaicin, the compound that gives chillies their 'burn'. Capsaicin seems to have a positive effect on blood cholesterol, and also works as an anticoagulant. The 'high' that some people experience when eating fiery chilli-spiked foods is a perfectly safe one. Some scientists theorize that in response to the discomfort produced by the chillies' 'burn', the brain releases endorphins, substances that, at high levels, can create a sensation of pleasure.

> ### Interesting!!
> Technically, chilli peppers are a fruit. Once dried, they are considered a spice.

CINNAMON

Cinnamon comes in 'quills', strips of bark rolled one in another. Like other powdered spices, cinnamon loses flavour quickly. Hence, it should be purchased in small quantities and kept away from light in airtight containers.

FROM THE LABS

Recent studies have determined that consuming as little as one-half teaspoon of cinnamon each day may reduce blood sugar, cholesterol, and triglyceride levels by as much as 20 per cent.

In a study at Copenhagen University, patients given half a teaspoon of cinnamon powder combined with one tablespoon of honey every morning before breakfast had significant relief from joint pains and arthritis after one week, and could walk without pain within one month.

It is mildly carminative and is used to treat nausea and flatulence. It is also used alone or in combination to treat diarrhoea. The cinnamaldehyde component is hypotensive and spasmolytic, and it increases peripheral blood flow. That's the reason this spice can help people with cold feet and hands, especially at night.

The essential oil of this herb is a potent antibacterial, anti-fungal, and uterine stimulant while the spice itself is a great source of manganese, fibre, iron and calcium.

> ### Interesting!!
> In the ancient world cinnamon was more precious than gold. Nero, Emperor of Rome in the first century AD, burned a year's supply of cinnamon on his wife's funeral pyre — an extravagant gesture meant to signify the depth of his loss.

CORIANDER

The fresh leaves of the plant are called cilantro and are used as a herb. The seeds are called coriander and are available both, whole and ground. The leaves have a distinctive fragrance.

The leaves of coriander are stimulant and tonic. They strengthen the stomach and promote its action, relieve flatulence, increase secretion and discharge of urine and reduce fever. They act as an aphrodisiac, help in the removal of catarrhal matter and phlegm from the bronchial tubes thereby counteracting any spasmodic disorders. Cilantro juice is highly beneficial in deficiencies of vitamin A, B1, B2, C and iron.

FROM THE LABS

Recent studies have supported its use as a stomach soother for both adults and colicky babies. Coriander contains an antioxidant that helps prevent animal fats from turning rancid. It has been shown to improve tummy troubles of all kinds, from indigestion to flatulence to diarrhoea. Cilantro and coriander seeds contain substances that kill certain bacteria and fungi, thereby preventing infections from developing in wounds.

Interesting!!

It is referred to in the Bible in the books of Exodus and Numbers, where the colour of 'manna' is compared to coriander.

CUMIN

This strong, heavy and warm spice commonly found and easily available has a spicy-sweet aroma. Ground cumin must be kept airtight, to retain its pungency. This spice should be used with restraint because it can exclude all the other flavours in a dish.

FROM THE LABS

Scientific studies have shown that oil in cumin helps reduce inflammation and eliminate fungus infections. The extract form has shown to be effective in regulating blood sugar levels, and stimulating bone marrow and immune cells.

Cumin is stomachic, diuretic, carminative, stimulant, astringent, and anti-spasmodic. It is supposed to increase lactation and reduce nausea in pregnancy. It has been shown to be effective in treating carpal tunnel syndrome, as well as diarrhoea, indigestion, and morning sickness. Cumin stimulates the appetite.

FENNEL

Fennel yields both a herb and a spice. All plant parts are edible – roots, stalks and leaves, with the spice coming from the dried seeds.

FROM THE LABS

Like many of its fellow spices, fennel contains its own unique combination of phytonutrients that give it a strong antioxidant activity. It helps to detoxify and remove waste material from the body. The major constituents of fennel are found in its volatile oil. This volatile oil has been shown to protect the liver from toxic chemical injury. It inhibits spasms in smooth muscles, such as those in the intestinal tract, and this is thought to contribute to fennel's use as a carminative (gas relieving and gastrointestinal tract cramp relieving agent).

Fennel is known to possess diuretic (increase in urine production), choleretic (increase in production of bile), pain-reducing, fever-reducing, and anti-microbial actions. The seeds and roots help to open obstructions of the liver, spleen and gall bladder, and to ease painful swellings.

MUSTARD

Three different species of mustard are grown for their seeds – white mustard, black mustard and brown mustard. The seed itself has no aroma while the flavour is sharp and fiery.

FROM THE LABS

Mustard seeds are a very good source of omega-3 fatty acids as well as calcium, dietary fibre, iron, manganese, magnesium, niacin, phosphorus, protein, selenium and zinc.

This small but powerful spice can increase your metabolic rate. It stimulates digestion, increasing saliva as much as eight times more than normal, reduces severity of asthma, decreases symptoms of rheumatoid arthritis, inhibits cancer cell growth, lowers high blood pressure, can prevent migraines and facilitates gastric juices improving your digestion.

Additionally it has four dynamic qualities: It is anti-bacterial, anti-fungal, anti-septic and has anti-inflammatory properties.

Interesting!!

Powdered mustard is usually made from white mustard seed and is often called mustard flour. When dry, it is as bland as cornstarch — mixed with cool water, its pungency emerges after a glucoside and an enzyme has a chance to combine in a chemical reaction.

PEPPER

This robust spice has an aromatic and pungent bouquet with a very pungent and fiery flavour. On a scale of hotness, black pepper scores an 8, white pepper is less pungent at 7, and green pepper is milder with a cleaner, fresher flavour and a score of 3 on the hotness scale. Whole peppercorns keep their flavour indefinitely but quickly lose aroma and heat after they have been grounded. They are very hard but are easily grounded in a peppermill.

FROM THE LABS

Peppercorns are stomachic, carminative, aromatic stimulant, antibacterial and diaphoretic (promoting sweat). They stimulate the taste buds causing reflex stimulation of gastric secretions, improving digestion, and treating gastro-intestinal upsets and flatulence.

This wonderful seasoning has demonstrated impressive antioxidant and anti-bacterial effects. Not only does it help you derive the maximum benefit from your food, the outer layer of the peppercorn stimulates the breakdown of fat cells, keeping you slim while giving you energy to burn.

Interesting!!

Soon after dawn on May 21, 1498, Vasco da Gama and his crew arrived at Calicut after the first direct sea voyage from Europe to Asia. If history's modern age has a beginning, this is it. And what did the men shout as they came ashore? 'For Christ and spices!'

TURMERIC

This colourful spice is an excellent detoxifier for the body. It purifies blood and cleanses intestines of bacteria. True wellness comes from good digestion, and this spice tops the list in making that possible. It corrects the disordered process of nutrition, and restores normalcy in the digestive system.

FROM THE LABS

'Curcumin' the main active Ingredient in this spice protects you from a host of age related disorders. It lowers cholesterol, protects the liver from toxins, boosts stomach defences against acid, reduces sugar in diabetes and has been shown to be active against Staphylococcus aureus (pus-producing infections).

Interesting!!

Its use dates back nearly 4000 years, to the Vedic culture in India where it was used as a culinary spice and had some religious significance. The name derives from the Latin 'terra merita' meaning 'meritorious earth' referring to the colour of ground turmeric which resembles a mineral pigment.

VANILLA

The flavouring comes from the seed pod, or the 'bean' of the vanilla plant. The prepared beans are very dark brown, slender and pleated. All beans contain thousands of tiny black seeds. Vanilla extract is also available and, if of good quality, is identical in flavour to the pods.

FROM THE LABS

Like many polyphenols found in plants, natural vanillin has antioxidant and anti-tumour activity. It is considered one of the most popular non-pungent spices – in actual fact it is one of the most widely used flavours in the world. Vanilla has always been held with high regard, as it was a spice used by the Spanish royalty. It has been used for stomachaches, to cure impotence, to exhilarate the brain, prevent sleep, to increase muscular energy, as an aphrodisiac and to help lower fever.

BEWARE

Substances called 'vanilla flavour' don't contain vanilla at all, being synthesized from eugenol (clove oil), waste paper pulp, coal tar or 'coumarin', found in the tonka bean, whose use is forbidden in several countries. Vanilla extract and vanilla flavour are two separate and distinct products.

Interesting!!

A good way to store whole vanilla is to bury it in rock candy. Use a jar with a tight fitting lid that will hold about a pound of rock candy, burying the bean so that no light can reach it. After 2-3 weeks, the granules will taste of vanilla and can be used in exotic blends or in other recipes, and the bean can be removed for other uses and returned to the rock candy after cleaning. Keep topping up the rock candy.

TOOLS OF HEALTH– VEGETABLES

INDIAN GOOSEBERRY

Amla enhances food absorption, balances stomach acid, fortifies the liver, nourishes the brain and mental functioning, supports the heart, strengthens the lungs, regulates elimination, enhances fertility, helps the urinary system, is good for the skin, promotes healthier hair, acts as a body coolant, flushes out toxins, increases vitality, strengthens the eyes, improves muscle tone, and it acts as an antioxidant. It is the panacea from the Indian subcontinent.

The fresh fruit contains more than 80 per cent water, protein, minerals, carbohydrates and fibre. Over the past centuries it has been used as and in remedies for fever, liver disorder, indigestion, anaemia, urinary problems, respiratory problems, cerebral, gastro and cardiovascular illnesses. Gooseberry lowers cholesterol levels also. It increases red blood cell production and strengthens teeth and nails.

FROM THE LABS

A study done in Japan by scientists at the Faculty of Pharmaceutical Sciences at Nagasaki University discovered through preliminary research that amla fruit extracts prevent the growth of cancerous cells. The cells that reacted best to the amla fruit extracts were the cells of the stomach, skin and womb. Along with these results and the powerful combination of antioxidant chemicals found in amla fruit, it is no wonder that this fruit is playing an important role in the fight against cancer. By co-relation, foods that prevent cancer are also the ones to build stronger immune systems.

BABY CORN

Baby corn can be found fresh, frozen, or canned in your local supermarket. The maximum nutrition and the type to use to increase immunity is the fresh variety. Baby corn contains substances called carotenoids, such as zeaxanthin and lutein. In "The 150 Healthiest Foods on Earth," Dr Jonny Bowden states that these two particular carotenoids promote eye health. You can help your children keep their eyesight strong by including this sweet and tender vegetable in their daily diet.

FASTER WOUND HEALING

Baby corn and other vegetables are natural sources of the mineral sodium which keeps the blood alkaline and vitamin C, or ascorbic acid. Vitamin C strengthens blood vessels, assisting in iron absorption and speeding the healing process of wounds.

FROM THE LABS

Baby corn is good source of a B vitamin called folate, or folic acid. Folate is used by the body to break down and synthesize amino acids from proteins. This process is necessary to build new cells, especially red blood cells. Baby corn also supplies other types of B vitamins such as thiamine, riboflavin and niacin. The B vitamins work together to digest and metabolize food. This vegetable is also a source of complex carbohydrates and protein. According to Washington State University, the more yellow the corn is, the more carotenoids it contains and thus, more useful as an immunity enhancer food.

BEETROOTS

This vegetable called beet, is a firm, clean, globe shaped vegetable with no soft wet areas. If still attached, it should have fresh, clean young leaves. Beetroots are characterized by dark purple skin and a distinctive purple flesh.

FROM THE LABS

Beets are high in potassium, folacin, and fibre. Their edible leaves offer protein, calcium, fibre, beta-carotene, vitamins A and C, and some B vitamins. Containing the powerful antioxidant betacyanin, which gives beetroot its deep red hue, this vegetable purifies the blood and has anti-carcinogenic properties. Research shows it boosts the body's natural defenses in the liver, regenerating immune cells. It also contains silica, vital for healthy skin, fingernails, ligaments, tendons and bones. Beetroot has liver, spleen, gall bladder and kidney cleansing properties. The iron contained in beetroot is organic and non-irritating and does not cause constipation. It is extremely rich in alkaline elements and beneficial for people who have acidosis.

Interesting!!

In pre-Christian times, the leaves of the beetroot were only eaten. Today, the root is used more often than the leaves since it stays fresher longer.

BELL PEPPERS

Bell peppers are like the Christmas ornaments of the vegetable world since they are beautifully shaped, glossy in appearance, and come in a variety of vivid colours such as green, red, yellow, orange, purple, brown and black. Also known as sweet peppers, they have a delightful, slightly watery crunch. Green and purple peppers have a slightly bitter flavour, while the red, orange and yellow ones are sweeter and almost fruity. Pimento and paprika are both prepared from red bell peppers.

COLOURFUL PROTECTION

Want to colour your life healthy? Brightly coloured bell peppers, whether green, red, orange or yellow, are rich sources of some of the best nutrients available. To begin, they are excellent sources of vitamin C and vitamin A, two very powerful antioxidants. These antioxidants work together to effectively neutralize free radicals, which can travel through the body causing huge amounts of damage to cells.

FROM THE LABS

Red peppers are one of the few foods that contain lycopene, a carotenoid whose consumption has been inversely correlated with prostate cancer and cancers of the cervix, bladder and pancreas. Consuming foods rich in beta-cryptoxanthin, an orange-red carotenoid found in highest amounts in red bell peppers, pumpkin, papaya, tangerines, etc. may significantly lower your risk of developing lung cancer.

This 'vegetable' contains vitamin B6 and folic acid. It has a protective effect against cataracts, possibly due to the vitamin C and beta-carotene content. Italian researchers compared the diets of hospital patients who had cataracts removed with patients who had not undergone the operation. Certain vegetables, including sweet peppers, reduced the cataract operation risk. The red variety of bell peppers also supply phytonutrients like lutein and zeaxanthin, which have been found to protect against macular degeneration, the main cause of blindness in the elderly.

Interesting!!

Christopher Columbus brought sweet peppers back to Europe where they quickly became a popular ingredient in Spanish cuisine.

BROCCOLI

The immunity building powers of this vegetable are phenomenal. Looking for a vitamin C fix? Make a beeline for broccoli. Are your potassium stores low? Partner up with broccoli. Is fibre on your shopping list? Bring home broccoli. Need an iron boost? Look no further than broccoli.

After recognizing broccoli's many attributes you can start to relish it for its lusty flavour.

Though most commercial markets sell only green broccoli, there are cultivars that produce purple and white broccoli. These are more common in Europe and so closely resemble cauliflower in appearance that they are easily confused.

SUPERHERO OF THE VEGETABLE KINGDOM

Broccoli's dark green colour is an indicator of its hearty carotene content. Though a bit on the bitter side, broccoli leaves are completely edible and also contain generous amounts of vitamin A. There is abundant folic acid and more bio-available calcium than pasteurized milk. Broccoli offers you 10 per cent of your daily iron requirement, and the vitamin C content helps the body to absorb the iron. A cup of broccoli actually fulfills your daily vitamin C requirement. With the good it can do you, this vegetable should make a frequent appearance at your dinner table.

Across the nutrition scale, broccoli contains all the nutrients mentioned above in addition to vitamins B1, B2, B3, B6, iron, magnesium, potassium, and zinc.

Most of the beta-carotene is stored in the florets. But don't jump too quickly. There's plenty of nutrition in those stems, such as extra calcium, iron, thiamine, riboflavin, niacin, and vitamin C. The darker colours of the florets, such as blue green, or purplish green contain more beta-carotene and vitamin C than those with lighter greens.

Because of its impressive nutritional profile that includes beta-carotene, vitamin C, calcium, fibre, and phytochemicals, specifically indoles and aromatic isothiocynates, broccoli and its kin may be responsible for boosting certain enzymes that help to detoxify the body. These enzymes help to prevent age from showing in your health by protecting you from age related disorders like cancer, diabetes, heart disease, osteoporosis, and high blood pressure.

No drugs required: Broccoli along with onions, carrots, and cabbage may also help to lower blood cholesterol. At the US Department of Agriculture's regional research center in Philadelphia, two researchers, Dr Peter Hoagland and Dr Philip Pfeffer, discovered these vegetables contain a certain pectin fibre called calcium pectate that binds to bile acids, holding more cholesterol in the liver and releasing less into the blood stream. They found broccoli equally as effective as some cholesterol lowering drugs.

Broccoli's wealth of the trace mineral, chromium, can be effective in preventing adult-onset diabetes in some people.

Interesting!!

Roman farmers called broccoli 'the five green fingers of Jupiter'.

CABBAGE

Common green cabbages have thick leaves, which are tightly wrapped to form a large dense head. The flavour of this versatile vegetable is strong and peppery.

FROM THE LABS

In its raw state, cabbage contains iron, calcium, and potassium. High marks are given for its vitamin C content. Cabbage is also high in vitamins B1, B2, and B3. Lengthy cooking tends to lower the nutritional value considerably.

Red cabbage is higher in fibre than green. It's also higher in vitamin C, calcium, iron, and potassium than its green cousin. Wrapped in a plastic bag and stored in the refrigerator, cabbage will keep up to three weeks. However, for its best flavour and nutrition, serve cabbage at its freshest. Include the core of the cabbage while using for any recipe. Many people toss it out, but it has the healthful nutrients and is a must for regenerative food pattern.

Researchers have learned that foods in the cabbage family inhibit the growth of breast, stomach, and colon cancer due to phytochemicals called indoles. These plant chemicals seem to produce anti-cancer enzymes. A University of Utah School of Medicine study on 600 men revealed that those who ate the most cruciferous vegetables had a much lower risk of colon cancer.

Interesting!!

A well known remedy for healing peptic ulcers is drinking cabbage juice. A medical study at Stanford University's School of Medicine gave thirteen ulcer patients five doses a day of cabbage juice. All were healed within seven to ten days with the vitamin U contained in the cabbage juice.

CARROT

A carrot a day ought to be added to the apple a day motto for its outstanding health benefits. The beta-carotene in carrots gets converted to vitamin A in your body. While animal foods contain vitamin A, fruits and vegetables contain only the vitamin's precursors – the carotenoids. One large raw carrot packs a whopping 20,253 IU of beta-carotene. Now that's a health aware person's delight! With 1 gram of protein and 2 grams of fibre, this crunchy treat has only 7 grams of carbohydrate and zero fat.

FROM THE LABS

Researchers at the USDA found that study participants who consumed 2 carrots a day were able to lower their cholesterol levels about 20 per cent due to a soluble fibre called calcium pectate.

Carrots are packed with nutrients. Raw carrots contain vitamins B1, B2, B3, B6 and offer 10.1 mcg of folic acid. You can supply your body with 233 mg of potassium from one large raw carrot that even contains vitamin C, iron, magnesium, and 19.4 mg of calcium. Additionally, the minerals – zinc, cobalt, fluorine, silicon, and chlorophyll make an appearance along with the amino acids – arganine, lysine, phenylanine, threonine, tryptophan, and valine. Potent antioxidants are among carrots' best features. These include the monoterpenes that protect against heart disease and cancer and polyacetylenes that inhibit tumour growth. The beta-carotene prevents cataract and premature aging.

Carrots contain a small amount of vitamin K, a fat soluble vitamin that helps with blood clotting and prevents the body from losing calcium loss through urination. On the sweetness scale among vegetables, while beets score the highest, carrots rank second with a sugar content of 7 per cent.

CAULIFLOWER

As an excellent source of vitamin C, and a very good source of manganese, cauliflower provides us with two core conventional antioxidants. But its antioxidant support extends far beyond the conventional nutrients into the realm of phytonutrients. Beta-carotene, beta-cryptoxanthin, caffeic acid, cinnamic acid, ferulic acid, quercetin, rutin, and kaempferol are among cauliflower's key antioxidant phytonutrients. This broad spectrum antioxidant support helps lower the risk of oxidative stress in our cells.

FROM THE LABS

There are several dozen studies linking cauliflower-containing diets to cancer prevention, particularly with respect to the following types of cancer: Bladder cancer, breast cancer, colon cancer, prostate cancer, and ovarian cancer. This connection between cauliflower and cancer prevention should not be surprising, since cauliflower provides special nutrient support for the immune system.

In research done at John Hopkins University in Baltimore, sulforaphane (found in cauliflower) lowered the occurrence of breast tumours in lab animals by almost 40 per cent. Toxins that would normally damage the cells and turn cancerous are swept out of the system by sulforaphane, preventing tumours before they begin.

CELERY

While most people associate celery with its prized stalks, its leaves, roots and seeds are also used as a food, seasoning and as a natural medicinal remedy. The stalks have a crunchy texture and a delicate, but mildly salty in taste. The stalks in the center are called the heart and are the most tender.

FROM THE LABS

Celery contains vitamin C and several other active compounds that promote health, including phthalides, which can help lower cholesterol, and coumarins, that may be useful in the prevention of malignant growths. Vitamin C rich foods like celery can reduce cold symptoms and support your immune system. The active compounds called phthalides, help relax the muscles around arteries and allow those vessels to dilate. With more space inside the arteries, the blood can flow at a lower pressure.

The seeds of celery's wild ancestors, which originated around the Mediterranean, were widely used as a diuretic. Modern science now understands how celery, which is rich in both potassium and sodium, the minerals most important for regulating fluid balance, stimulates urine production, and helps to rid the body of excess fluid.

Interesting!!

The initial mention of the beneficial properties of celery leaves dates back to ninth century B.C., when celery made an appearance in the Odyssey, the famous epic by the Greek poet, Homer.

CUCUMBER

Technically, cucumber is a fruit because it contains seeds to reproduce, but typically they are grouped with vegetables due to their use.

FROM THE LABS

Cucumbers are about 95 per cent water. They are cool and moist due to their high water content. Cucumbers are high in potassium and fibre with moderate amounts of Vitamins A and C, as well as folic acid, phosphorus, and magnesium. This refreshing 'vegetable' contains compounds called 'sterols' which have been shown to lower cholesterol. The heaviest concentration of sterols is in the skin of the cucumber, so it's best not to remove the peel before eating. They are great for digestion and exert a cleansing effect on the bowel.

Interesting!!

'Cool as a cucumber' isn't just a catchy phrase. The inner temperature of a cucumber can be up to 20 degrees cooler than the outside air. No wonder these are such a summer time favourite!

FRENCH BEANS

Green beans, also known as string beans are one of the only few varieties of beans that are eaten fresh. They are picked while still immature and the inner bean is just beginning to form. In comparison to the dried bean varieties, the green bean offers less protein but more fibre and other nutrients. Their fibre can help promote a healthy colon because of its ability to bind to disease-causing toxins, removing them from the body before they can harm colon cells. Green beans have strong anti-inflammatory effects which make it effective in diseases where inflammation takes place, besides being helpful for menstruating girls and for teens who are at risk of iron deficiency.

FROM THE LABS

It's impossible to describe the potential nutritional benefits of green beans and not mention bone health. It has a rich concentration of silicon, vitamin K, calcium, magnesium and phosphorus and each of these nutrients has been shown to play a key role in bone health. In the case of vitamin K, green beans are an excellent source of this nutrient and provide an unusually great amount of vitamin K. In the case of silicon, not only do green beans provide a valuable amount of this mineral, but they also appear to do so in a way that is easier for the body to absorb.

Because of their rich green colour, we don't always think about French beans as providing us with important amounts of colourful pigments like carotenoids. But they do! Recent studies have confirmed the presence of lutein, beta-carotene, violaxanthin, and neoxanthin in them. In some cases, the presence of these carotenoids in green beans is comparable to their presence in other carotenoid rich vegetables like carrots and tomatoes. The only reason you don't see these carotenoids is because of the concentrated chlorophyll content of green beans.

GARLIC

Garlic's secret armory consists of more than 33 active sulphur-containing substances that battle with enemies such as bacteria, viruses, and fungi. Some of the more familiar compounds are allicin, alliin, cycroalliin, and diallyldisulphide. Allicin, garlic's warrior against bacteria and inflammation, is also the culprit behind its offensive odour. Garlic's antibiotic effect is attributed to alliin, the sulphur-containing amino acid responsible for the manufacture of allicin.

EQUIVALENT TO THE STRONGEST DRUGS

To demonstrate garlic's amazing strength, imagine that one milliliter of raw garlic juice can be compared to a milligram of streptomycin or sixty micrograms of penicillin. Garlic is one of nature's strongest, most complex, broad spectrum antibacterial agents. Tests show that garlic kills or cripples at least 72 infectious bacteria found during diarrhoea, dysentery, botulism and tuberculosis among other diseases.

Garlic's sulphur containing compounds offer many health benefits including the ability to regulate blood sugar metabolism, stimulate and detoxify the liver, and stimulate the nervous system and blood circulation.

Garlic's ability to lower serum cholesterol is attributed to diallyldisulphide oxide. The high level of selenium in garlic is believed to prevent sticky platelets and ward off atherosclerosis and clot formation in the arteries.

Those who suffer from allergies usually find that garlic strengthens their immune system and reduces the effect of allergens. One of garlic's non-sulphur components, a flavone called quercetin, may be responsible for stabilizing mast cells at the onset of asthma and allergy conditions. Mast cells, part of our immune system, help the body recognize potential invading organisms. Garlic also contains phenolic properties that provide antioxidant effects. Garlic has the surprising ability to retain its antioxidant properties for up to six months after it is harvested.

Garlic is a mini storehouse of minerals. Manganese, copper, iron, zinc, sulphur, calcium, aluminum, chlorine, and selenium are all part of the minerals contained in garlic. One hundred grams, or 3 1/2 ounces, of fresh garlic will supply you with:

Copper – 0.30 mg
Iron – 1.7 mg
Manganese – 1.12 mg
Phosphorous – 153 mg

Selenium – 14.2 mg
Zinc – 1.16 mg

LIFT YOURSELF

Investigators testing garlic have noticed that garlic eaters experience a decided lift in mood – have a greater feeling of well being. They experienced measurably less fatigue, anxiety, sensitivity, agitation and irritability. This mood lifting bonus of garlic is important and in sharp contrast to the adverse side effects of many pharmaceutical drugs.

Interesting!!

In support of garlic, the ancient Egyptian medical papyri, Codex Elsers, dated about 1500 BC, contained 22 formulas for medicinal remedies prescribing garlic as a cure for heart disease, worms, and tumours. The Egyptian remedies may have actually originated as early as 3500 BC before written forms existed.

GINGER

Ginger is most commonly known for its effectiveness as a digestive aid. By increasing the production of digestive fluids and saliva, it strengthens your digestion helping you extract more nutrients from your food without any gas pains, diarrhoea or stomach cramping. Ginger root has been found to be even more effective than pharmaceutical drugs in curbing motion sickness, without causing drowsiness. This vegetable's anti-inflammatory properties help relieve pain and reduce inflammation associated with arthritis, rheumatism and muscle spasms. Its therapeutic properties effectively stimulate circulation of the blood, removing toxins from the body, cleansing the bowels and kidneys, and nourishing the skin.

Interesting!!

It takes its name from the Sanskrit word stringa-vera, which means 'with a body like a horn', since it is shaped like antlers.

GREEN PEAS

Peas flaunt twice the protein of most vegetables, so they're the ideal substitute for fattier protein fare, providing an excellent strategy for controlling your fat intake. Green peas, like dried peas, are legumes, except they're eaten before they mature. As with all legumes, they're chock-full of nutrients. Peas have lutein, the carotenoid with a proven record of helping to reduce the risk of age-related macular degeneration and cataract, and maintain your immune system. Green peas are one of the important foods to include in your children's diet if they often feel fatigued and sluggish. That is because they provide nutrients that help support the energy producing cells and systems of the body.

FROM THE LABS

Green peas provide nutrients that are important for maintaining bone health. They are a very good source of vitamin K, some of which our bodies convert into K2, which activates osteocalcin, the major non-collagen protein in bone. Osteocalcin anchors calcium molecules inside of the bone. Therefore, without enough vitamin K2, osteocalcin levels are inadequate and bone mineralization is impaired.

Peas are a very good source of thiamine – vitamin B1 and a good source of vitamin B6, riboflavin – vitamin B2 and niacin – vitamin B3, all of which are nutrients that are necessary for carbohydrate, protein and lipid metabolism.

ICEBERG LETTUCE

Christopher Columbus was said to have brought lettuce to the new world. 'Crisp head' was what lettuce was called originally until the 1920's when transporters began shipping it beneath ice to keep it fresh, which is how it came to be known as iceberg lettuce. This variety of lettuce is preferred over most other types of lettuce due to its moist crispiness. While it's true that most darker greens are richer in nutrients, iceberg lettuce is still a very healthy choice.

The usual green leaf lettuce tends to be somewhat bitter, and due to the high water content of iceberg lettuce, mixing the two helps eliminate the bitterness of the leaf lettuce.

FROM THE LABS

Iceberg lettuce is low in saturated fat and there is zero cholesterol in it. It is also a good source of iron and vitamin A, B6, C and K. It is a good source of dietary fibre, which is important to maintain good overall health. Nutritional benefits of iceberg lettuce are enhanced due to the folate present in it, and the fact that it contains traces of omega fatty acids, which help in maintaining the heart and brain healthy.

LEMONS

The juice is more or less 40-50 per cent of the mass of the lemon, is yellow-greenish in colour, sour in taste and its chemical composition includes 5-7 per cent citric acid, free and combined organic acids, 2-3 per cent sugars, nitrogenous substances and vitamins (especially vitamin C or ascorbic acid).

FROM THE LABS

When considering the electromagnetic properties of food, it has been discovered that all foods are considered cationic with the exception of fresh, raw lemon juice. This is similar to our saliva which is anionic. The negatively charged lemon juice alkalinizes the body keeping our muscles and cells supple and young. An acidic system will always tend towards premature aging and disorders. It should be noted that pasteurized and packaged lemon juice is cationic and, therefore, ineffective as a health remedy.

THE COMMON YET POWERFUL LEMON

It prevents sepsis (the presence of pathogenic bacteria) or putrefaction (decomposition of tissues). It is also anti-scorbutic, which means a remedy to prevent disease and assists in cleansing the system of impurities. By consuming lemon juice regularly, the bowels are aided in eliminating wastes more efficiently thus, controlling constipation and diarrhoea.

Lemon is a wonderful stimulant for the liver, and a dissolvent of uric acid and other poisons. It liquefies bile, and assists fat metabolism. Sufferers of chronic rheumatism and gout will benefit by taking lemon juice. Also those who have a tendency to bleed, have uterine haemorrhages, etc. are also benefitted by it. In pregnancy, it will help to build bone in the child. As a food, owing to its potassium content, it will nourish the brain and nerve cells. Its calcium builds up the bony structure and makes healthy teeth. Its magnesium, in conjunction with calcium, has an important part to play in the formation of albumin in the blood.

In 'the plan' described for regeneration, the purpose of using lemon is:

1. To provide a natural strengthening agent to the liver enzymes when they are too dilute.
2. The liver can make more enzymes out of fresh lemon juice than any other food element.
3. The lemon helps fix oxygen and calcium in the liver.

Interesting!!

Lemon is one of the only foods on the planet that has more anions than cations in its atomic structure.

ONIONS

In Chinese medicine, globe onions are said to calm the liver, moisten the intestines, and benefit the lungs. Raw onions are prescribed for constipation, for lowering high blood pressure, and for healing wounds or ulcers of the skin. Spring onions, or scallions are used to induce sweating.

FROM THE LABS

Onions and other members of the family Liliaceae (garlic, leek, green onion, etc.) contain tens of flavonoids, complexes that prevent cardiovascular disease. These substances lower blood cholesterol, liquefy the blood, and prevent hardening of the arteries. Some health studies have shown raw onions to be effective in lowering overall cholesterol while raising HDLs, the good cholesterol. Additionally, onions kill infectious bacteria, they help to control blood sugar, and aid in dissolving blood clots.

Asthma sufferers can also benefit from a hearty dose of onions. Researchers have discovered a sulphur compound contained in onions that can prevent the biochemical chain reaction leading to asthma attacks.

Interesting!!

Of all foods in the plant kingdom, onions set the record for the most frequent appearance in ancient Egyptian art.

RADISH LEAVES

Radishes belong to the mustard family which explains their sharp taste. You may have seen them in white or red colour, but it can be found in black, purple, rose and even lavender. Radish is one of the richest sources of iron, calcium and sodium among all the common vegetables. The leaves are also eaten and used as salad, chutney, in sprouts, or in yoghurts. Not only is the radish a solid source of fibre and roughage aiding in digestion, but it also contains many detoxifying characteristics.

FROM THE LABS

Radishes are quite high in ascorbic acid and folic acid. They are also a rich source of potassium, riboflavin and magnesium. Radish is generally a diuretic, but it also aids in the treatment of inflammation and eases urination. Radishes also contain a good source of lycopene, which scientific studies have shown to drastically reduce the risk of certain types of cancer. Additionally, many skin disorders have been treated with this vegetable as it appears to help retain moisture in the skin, and also acts as a productive disinfectant.

Interesting!!

In Greece, radishes were so highly valued that imitations of them were made of gold.

SWEET CORN

Many of you know that as a vegetable, corn can be served in a variety of delicious ways. Very few people are aware of the fact that corn is a highly nutritious food item which can provide numerous health benefits.

A REJUVENATING FOOD

It has been found that consuming corn daily can help in the strengthening of hair follicles due to its powerful antioxidants like vitamin C and lycopene. These also help in keeping one's skin healthy and smooth. You should make it a point to add corn to your child's diet to provide health with taste.

FROM THE LABS

Corn is rich in a variety of essential nutrients like vitamin B1 which is useful in the metabolism of carbohydrates; vitamin B5 which helps in psychological functions; vitamin C; and is also rich in folate which helps in the generation of new cells. It has been found that eating corn can enhance mental and psychological functions due to its high content of thiamine. Moreover, the consumption of corn can also help in the prevention of fatigue as it contains beta-carotene which increases the supply of haemoglobin in the body.

TOMATO

As a health promoting vegetables, tomatoes can be placed on the highest pedestal because they contain the antioxidant lycopene, noted for its ability to reduce the risk of malignant development in the body.

Tomatoes also contain vitamin C and carotenoids, beta-carotene being one of the most familiar antioxidants. These offer protection from free radicals that cause premature aging, cancer, heart disease, and cataract. As they are loaded with antioxidants and are high in potassium, tomatoes are one of the healthiest 'vegetables' you can add to your regular food patterns. It is to be noted that most of the benefits of the antioxidants are from RAW tomato and not the cooked version.

Interesting!!

The French loved them and referred to them as 'love apples'. In Germany they were revered as 'apples of paradise'.

TURNIPS

These are a 'starch' vegetable, but contain only one third the amount as compared to an equal amount of potatoes. Turnips have a little sweet and refreshing taste. Usually the smaller ones taste better because the big turnips are old and more hard to eat.

Turnips provide an excellent source of vitamin C, fibre, folic acid, manganese, pantothenic acid, and copper. They also offer a very good source of thiamine, potassium, niacin, and magnesium. In addition, they are a good source of vitamin B6 and E, folic acid, and riboflavin. Turnip greens are more nutrition dense than the root. The greens provide an excellent source of vitamins A, B6, C, E, folic acid, calcium, copper, fibre and manganese.

From the labs: Excellent for the lungs and disorders related to it. Children with asthma, bronchitis, and adult smokers should eat turnips to help their body be healthier, cleanse the excessive phlegm, and alleviate the side effects of smoking. Children who play sports can build greater stamina and endurance levels by eating this vegetable. They will develop stronger lung capacity.

YOUR POT-POURRI

ALMONDS

A high-fat food that's good for your health? That's not an oxymoron, its almonds. Almonds are high in monounsaturated fats, the same type of health-promoting fats as are found in olive oil. They contain no cholesterol since they are a plant food and only animal sourced foods contain cholesterol. To go beyond this, eating almonds can lower your cholesterol. A study published in the British Journal of Nutrition indicates that when foods independently known to lower cholesterol, such as almonds, are combined in a healthy way of eating, the beneficial effects are cumulative.

Almonds are high in protein, containing about 20 per cent of it. One ounce contains 12 per cent of our daily protein needs. Vitamin E, considered a powerful antioxidant with cancer fighting qualities, is plentiful in almonds. The flavonoids found in almond skins team up with the vitamin E found in their meat to more than double the antioxidant punch either delivers when administered separately, shows a study published in the Journal of Nutrition.

They're also high in magnesium, having even more than spinach. Almonds are abundant in phosphorus, which is good for bones and teeth. They are higher in calcium than all other nuts. If you are pregnant, almonds can be a nutritious way of preventing certain birth defects because of their high folic acid content.

Almond's healthy fats may help you lose weight: A study published in the International Journal of Obesity and Related Metabolic Disorders that included 65 overweight and obese adults suggests that an almond enriched low energy diet (which is high in monounsaturated fats) can help overweight individuals shed pounds more effectively than a low energy diet high in complex carbohydrates.

Interesting!!

Almonds along with dates, grapes, and olives were among the earliest cultivated foods, probably before 3,000 BC. Almonds and pistachios are the only nuts mentioned in the bible.

BASIL

The taste of sweet basil is far less pungent than the permeating, heady aroma of the freshly picked leaves would suggest. Thus large quantities can be used with safety. Dried sweet basil leaves are quite different from the fresh, and although the fragrant, fresh smelling top notes or tender leaves disappear upon drying, a concentration of volatile oils in the cells of the dehydrated leaves give a pungent clove and allspice bouquet.

FROM THE LABS

Basil has a powerful essential oil that contains methyl chavicol. Fresh leaves contain folic acid, and dried basil is a good source of potassium, iron and calcium. The essential oil obtained from this plant also contains camphor.

The leaves of tulsi plant are a nerve tonic and also sharpen memory. They promote the removal of catarrhal matter and phlegm from the bronchial tube. The leaves strengthen the stomach. Its strong taste promotes the production of saliva, letting the body digest food properly, and assist you in keeping healthy.

Basil leaves are regarded as an 'adaptogen' or anti-stress agent. Recent studies have shown that the leaves afford significant protection against stress. Even healthy people can chew 12 leaves of basil, twice a day, to prevent stress. It purifies blood and helps prevent several common elements.

BARLEY GRAIN

A diet containing barley grain is one of the safest in terms of grain allergies. Barley is known to be gentle on the intestines and cooling for the entire digestive system. The fibre in barley helps promote digestion and reduces the risk of colon cancer. Like all whole grain products, barley can help keep blood pressure low and reduce the risk of type 2 diabetes when consumed regularly. It is more effective at regulating insulin and glucose responses than whole oats. When consumed as a part of a diet containing other whole grains, barley can contribute to a reduced risk of obesity, anaemia, constipation, headaches and migraines.

Barley's amazing properties make it no surprise that this grain has endured for millennia. But what is striking is the fact that people have been slow to embrace this grain as they have wheat, corn, rice, and oats. Fortunately, as new research unveils more and more ways that barley can be a healthful addition to your diet, it will become a more pervasive staple to your family's diet.

FROM THE LABS

Scientific research done on this grain has shown its intake to help you maintain overall health in the long term. Barley grains are rich in protein, vitamins, minerals and amino acids, which are essentials for your child's health. Most importantly, barley is one of the richest sources of both soluble and insoluble fibre. Insoluble fibre aids in proper excretion of waste products in the body; on the other hand, soluble fibre (aka beta glucan) mixes with liquids, binds to fatty substances and allows them to leave the body.

BROWN CHICK PEAS

This grain is one of the good sources of proteins for vegetarians and much liked by children. Combined with a whole grain such as whole wheat protein, they provide an adequate amount of protein comparable to that of meat, or dairy foods without the dangers.

Brown chick peas, also known as garbanzos are an excellent source of the trace mineral manganese, which is an essential co-factor in a number of enzymes important in energy production and antioxidant defenses. Just one cup of garbanzo beans supplies 84.5 per cent of the daily value for this mineral.

FROM THE LABS

Brown chick peas can boost your children's energy because of their high iron content. This is particularly important for menstruating teens and growing children.

Its soluble fibre helps stabilize blood sugar levels. If you have insulin resistance, hypoglycaemia or diabetes, beans like garbanzos can help balance blood sugar levels while providing steady, slow burning energy. The carbohydrate in them is broken down and digested slowly. This is also helpful for weight loss in obese children as it controls the appetite.

BROWN RICE

Brown rice is also known as unpolished rice and is rich in many vital nutrients. The rice consumed in most of the households is the white rice in which nutrients such as vitamin B and E are missing. Magnesium, potassium and iron are also missing in white rice. Shifting from white rice to brown rice can help your children in eating a balanced diet and also in gaining the essential nutrients such as Vitamin B and iron.

Brown rice is an excellent source of fibre and is favourable for the digestive system. It helps in the bowel movement and is good for curing constipation. It is useful in keeping the body feeling satiated.

FROM THE LABS

Medical researches carried out have shown that the fibre content in brown rice aids in keeping blood cholesterol levels in check. Research has also shown it in helping to keep blood sugar in control. It has been found to be beneficial for the treatment of asthma. It has also been found to contain anti-inflammatory compounds, which help in reducing breathlessness and wheezing in asthma.

CHICKEN

The health benefits of eating chicken are enormous. It is a rich source of a variety of essential nutrients and vitamins, which assist in strengthening the immune system of the body. Chicken is also reputed to be one of the safest meats available, as it is least associated with any side effects of consumption. It is a very good source of lean, high quality protein essential for growth and development.

FROM THE LABS

Chicken is a rich source of niacin, a B-vitamin that protects the body against cancer. A deficiency of niacin can be directly associated with genetic (DNA) damage. Around 72 per cent of the daily niacin requirement of the body can be fulfilled by a four-ounce serving. The trace mineral selenium found in good quantities in chicken is an essential component required by many major metabolic pathways, which includes thyroid hormone metabolism, anti-oxidant defense systems, and the immune function of the body.

Chicken meat is a good source of phosphorus, which is an essential mineral for the maintenance of teeth and bones, and also ensures healthy functioning of the kidneys, liver and the central nervous system.

COCONUT

Researchers have known for quite some time that the secret to health and weight loss associated with the coconut is related to the length of the fatty acid chains contained in coconut oil. These medium chain fatty acids are different from the common, longer chain fatty acids found in other plant based oils. Most vegetable oils are composed of longer chain fatty acids, or triglycerides

(LCTs). LCTs are typically stored in the body as fat, while MCTs are burned for energy. MCTs burn up quickly in the body. They are a lot like adding kindling to a fireplace, rather than a big damp log.

FROM THE LABS

Coconut is nature's richest source of MCTs. Not only do MCTs raise the body's metabolism, but they have special health giving properties as well. The most predominant MCT in coconut, for example, is lauric acid. Lipid researcher Dr Jon Kabara states, "Never before in the history of man is it so important to emphasize the value of lauric oils. The medium-chain fats in coconut are similar to fats in mother's milk and have similar nutriceutical effects."

The medium chain fatty acids and monoglycerides found primarily in coconut and mother's milk have miraculous healing power. Outside of a human mother's breast milk, coconut is nature's most abundant source of lauric acid and medium chain fatty acids.

CURRY LEAF

Curry plant is widely used for its culinary and medicinal properties.

FROM THE LABS

Curry leaves improve the functioning of the stomach and small intestine and promote their action. They improve the quality of digestive juices secreted during digestion. Their action starts with intake. Their smell, taste and visual impression initiates salivary secretion and initiates the peristaltic wave, which is the first step in good digestion. They are mildly laxative and thus can tackle multiple digestive problems caused by food intake. The chemical composition of the plant defines the aroma and the taste.

Interesting!!

A fully grown curry tree can yield nearly 100 kg of leaves each year.

EXTRA VIRGIN OLIVE OIL

Nutritional scientist Dr Joanna McMillan Price demonstrated at the recent World Congress on Oils and Fats the health benefits of extra virgin olive oil. He focused on how the Mediterranean diet, long touted as one of the world's healthiest, has been shown to assist in weight loss, is associated with low risk heart disease and certain cancers, and has been shown to reduce blood pressure in northern European men. One of the main ingredients and the main source of (monounsaturated) fats in the Mediterranean diet is extra virgin olive oil.

Its content of antioxidants, vitamins and nutrients protect you against illnesses, promotes healthy digestion, balances the fatty acids in the body, and prevents gallstone formation.

FROM THE LABS

Now, a team of researchers, including one with the Agricultural Research Service (ARS), has found that phenolic components in olive oil actually modify genes that are involved in the inflammatory response. ARS is the principal intramural scientific research agency of the US Department of Agriculture (USDA).

The study, published recently in Biomed Central (BMC) Genomics, was done by a multi-institute group of researchers headed by Francisco Perez-Jimenez with the University of Cordoba, Spain. Among the researchers was ARS computational biologist– Laurence Parnell, with the Nutrition and Genomics Laboratory at the Jean Mayer USDA Human Nutrition Research Center on Aging (HNRCA) at Tufts University in Boston, Massacheusets.

For the study, the researchers fed 20 volunteers—who had metabolic syndrome—with two virgin olive oil-based breakfasts, one at a time, after a six-week 'washout' period.

Metabolic syndrome is a prevalent condition often characterized as having a combination of abdominal obesity, high triglycerides, high blood pressure and poor blood sugar control, all of which increase risk for heart disease and diabetes.

All volunteers consumed the same low fat, carbohydrate rich 'background' diet during both study phases. The researchers tracked the expression of more than 15,000 human genes in blood cells during the after-meal period. The results indicated that 79 genes are turned down and 19 are turned up by the high-phenolic-content olive oil. Many of those genes have been linked to obesity, high blood-fat levels, type 2 diabetes and heart disease. Importantly, several of the turned down genes are known promoters of inflammation, so those genes may be involved in 'cooling off' inflammation that often accompanies metabolic syndrome.

The researchers concluded that the results shed light on a molecular basis for reduced disease risk among people living in Mediterranean countries where virgin olive oil is the main source of dietary fats.

TYPES OF OLIVE OIL

1. **Regular or Pure Olive Oil**
   Regular or pure olive oil has been chemically refined and filtered to neutralize both undesirable strong tastes and acid content. It is of lower quality and usually the least expensive.

2. **Virgin**

    Virgin means the olive oil was produced without any chemical additives, so it contains no refined oil. It has an acidity that's less than 2 per cent, so it tastes better. Virgin refers to the fact that the olive oil has been less handled or manipulated during processing.

3. **Extra Virgin**

    Extra virgin olive oil comes from the first press only and is the highest quality olive oil with perfect flavour, aroma, and balanced acidity. This oil is less processed than virgin olive oil and is very delicate in flavour. It's perfect for salad dressings, marinades, and for dipping bread.

4. **Cold Pressed Olive Oil**

    Cold pressed olive oil is an unregulated label description. Back when olive oil was pressed the second time using hot water and steam to extract the last drop, the heat during the second pressing took away the delicate flavours. Today, premium olive oil is cold pressed, which means the olive paste is gently warmed to room temperature to avoid losing taste and pressing is done in winter, when it's cold, to further retain flavour.

    My opinion is that the best olive oil you can buy is organic cold pressed, extra virgin olive oil. That's what I personally use.

GREEN MUNG BEANS

These much loved beans may be a humble food but is actually a nutritional powerhouse that can be defined as a super food. These beans from the legume family are rich in protein, vitamin C, folic acid, iron, zinc, potassium, magnesium, copper, manganese, phosphorus and thiamine. When sprouted, mung beans contain vitamin C that is not found in the bean itself.

Because of the wide range of nutrients contained in these beans, they offer a whole host of health benefits for the immune system, the metabolism, the heart and other organs, cell growth, protection against free radicals, and diseases such as cancer and diabetes.

FROM THE LABS

The folic acid contained in mung beans contributes to normal cell growth, helps in the metabolism of proteins, is essential for the formation of red blood cells, and for healing processes in the body. Another B vitamin, thiamine, is needed to ensure that the nervous system functions properly. It is also important for releasing energy from carbohydrates. Manganese is a trace mineral that is key for energy production and antioxidant defenses. It is also necessary for the metabolism of carbohydrates, fats, and proteins, and can be helpful for the brain and nerves.

Magnesium helps the veins and arteries to relax, lessening resistance and improving the flow of blood, oxygen, and nutrients throughout the body.

The body requires copper in order to absorb iron, and copper is also involved in the metabolism of protein. Potassium is necessary for maintaining the acid-alkaline balance in the blood for muscle contraction, and a normal heart beat. Zinc is a well known immune system booster and aids healing processes in the body, growth, and tissue repair.

HONEY

It is an organic, natural sugar alternative with no additives that is easy on the stomach, versatile in usage and has an indefinite shelf-life. There are as many flavours of honey as there are flowers, since the flavour of the honey is directly influenced by the type of nectar gathered by the bees from various floral sources.

FROM THE LABS

Honey is composed of sugars like glucose, fructose and minerals like magnesium, potassium, calcium, sodium chlorine, sulphur, iron and phosphate. It contains vitamins B1, B2, C, B6, B5 and B3 all of which change according to the qualities of the nectar and pollen. Besides the above minerals, copper, iodine, and zinc exist in it in small quantities. Several kinds of hormones are also present in it.

It also has different phytochemicals that kill viruses, bacteria, and fungus making it a good antiseptic. There is evidence that honey diluted in water will help with your stomachaches and dehydration. Because sugar molecules in honey can convert into other sugars (for example, fructose to glucose), honey is easily digested by the most sensitive stomachs, despite its high acid content. It helps kidneys and intestines to function better.

Honey rapidly diffuses through the blood. When accompanied by mild water, it can circulate in the bloodstream in 7 minutes. Its free sugar molecules make the brain function better since the brain is the largest consumer of sugar, hence reducing fatigue. In addition, it helps in cleansing the blood and has positive effects in regulating and facilitating blood circulation. It also functions as a protection against capillary problems and arteriosclerosis.

Interesting!!

Its 'magical' properties and versatility has given honey a significant part in history. Its name comes from the English 'hunig', and it was the first and most widespread sweetener used by man.

LEMON GRASS

Lemon grass is native to India. It is widely used as a herb in Asian cuisine. It has a citrus flavour and can be dried and powdered, or used fresh. Citral, an essential oil also found in lemon peel, is the constituent responsible for its taste and aroma.

Lemon grass is also known as 'gavati chaha' in Marathi language (gavat-grass; chaha-tea) is used as an addition to tea, and in preparations like 'kadha' which is a traditional herbal 'soup' against cough, cold, etc. It has many beneficial properties including rejuvenating the body due to which it has been used in different cultures across the world.

FROM THE LABS

Studies have shown lemon grass to contain anti-bacterial and anti-fungal properties. It helps to detoxify the liver, pancreas, kidney, bladder and the digestive tract. Besides these it helps boost the immune system, reduces uric acid, cholesterol, excess fats; It helps alleviate indigestion and gastroenteritis,

Lemon grass assists in toning the muscle and tissues, reduce blood pressure, and improves blood circulation. To keep you looking young and in shape, you will be like a celebrity, this grass helps reduce cellulite and improves the skin by reducing acne and pimples. As a stress buster, it acts as a sedative for the central nervous system calming you after your work.

Interesting!!

In 2006, a research team from the Ben Gurion University in Israel found that lemon grass (cymbopogoncitratus) caused apoptosis (programmed cell death) in malignant cancer cells. According to the research team, citral is the substance that causes the cancer cells to kill themselves.

MINT

Mint is well known for its ability to soothe the digestive tract and reduce the severity and length of stomachaches. In addition, exotic blends made from it have shown great promise at easing the discomfort associated with irritable bowel syndrome, and even at slowing the growth of many of the most harmful bacteria and fungi. The well documented anti-fungal properties of this refreshing herb are thought to play a role in the treatment of asthma and many allergic conditions as well. Mint is carminative, stimulative, stomachic, diaphoretic and anti-spasmodic. It is a general pick-me-up, good for colds, flu and fevers.

> ### Interesting!!
> Ancient Hebrews scattered mint on their synagogue floors so that each footstep would raise its fragrance. Ancient Greeks and Romans rubbed tables with mint before their guests arrived for its sweet aroma.

MOTH BEANS

Most of the commotion that beans are generating in the scientific community has to do with the fact that they are showing to provide protection from many of the most feared and lethal diseases plaguing the world today. They actually contain a wider variety of healthy nutrients than most foods. These nutrients work together on several key areas of the body promoting total health. Moth beans also happen to be good sources of complete proteins, which is rare in plants.

Studies done in universities have shown that eating beans offer the body valuable sources of ready energy that it can burn quickly and effectively. Because of this, moth beans are a super food for children.

FROM THE LABS

Associated with carbohydrates and gas, current studies have done a wonderful job of increasing our understanding of this plentiful food and revealed it to be packed with important nutrition. Michigan State University has performed studies that indicate 'dry' beans are the healthiest. Most beans contain similar nutrients, but it is generally thought that the best are lima beans, mung beans and moth beans. It is recommended that you get about three cups of beans per week into your child's diet to achieve the best health results, but even as little as a cup per week can help you achieve impressive results!

MUNNAKKA

Munakka are dried grapes, also known as a variety of raisins. The word raisin dates back to middle English and is a loanword from old French; in old French, raisin means 'grape'. Seedless varieties include the Sultana and Flame while the ones with seeds include munakkas. They are typically sun-dried, but may also be 'water-dipped' or dehydrated. Mini raisins are much darker in colour and have a tart, tangy flavour.

Munakkas contain high amounts of iron and vitamins needed by the body. As a result it assists children with anaemia through increasing haemoglobin in the blood. It is also helpful in treating other diseases of the blood that are caused by chronic fevers and inflammation.

FROM THE LABS

These delicious dried grapes have been the object of phytonutrient research primarily for their unique phenol content which shows tremendous antioxidant activity. The total antioxidant activity of many fruits and vegetables has been found to be exactly parallel to their total phenol content and raisins take their place in this list right at the top.

They are also an excellent source of boron, a trace mineral. Studies have shown boron to provide protection against osteoporosis. It reproduces many of the positive effects of oestrogen therapy in menopausal women. Munakkas, despite being sweet and sticky, not only do not cause cavities and gum disease, but actually promote oral health. The phytonutrients in them, specifically oleanolic acid are effective in killing bacteria found in cavities and periodontal dental disease.

Interesting!!

When most fruits are dried, they keep their same name, but not the grape. The dried form of the grape, revered throughout history, has its own unique name – the raisin. And each type of raisin has its own unique name.

OATS

Oatmeal in any form is a good way to meet part of the recommendation to eat whole grains each day. It is a known source of nutrients that can provide proven benefits on satiety and gastrointestinal health. Oats contain an ingredient called beta-glucan that supports the immune system.

FROM THE LABS

In laboratory studies reported, beta-glucan significantly enhanced the human immune system's response to bacterial infection. Beta-glucan not only helps neutrophils (the most abundant type of non-specific immune cell) navigate to the site of an infection more quickly, it also enhances their ability to eliminate the bacteria they find there.

According to one of the studies conducted by the Department of Surgery at Rhode Island Hospital and Brown University, study leader Jonathan Reichner concluded that priming neutrophils with beta-glucan helps these immune defenders quickly locate the bacterial mother lode within an infected tissue. And this more rapid response to infection results in faster microbial clearance and healing.

Since our non-specific immune defenses are the body's first strike force against invading pathogens, giving your kids a bowl of oats may boost their immune response in addition to their morning energy levels.

PREVENTING CHILDHOOD ASTHMA

In another path breaking study done by researchers from the Dutch National Institute of Public Health and the Environment, Utrecht University a co-relation was found between whole grains like oats and childhood asthma. They assessed the children's (aged 8-13 years) consumption of a range of foods including fish, fruits, vegetables, dairy and whole grain products. Data on asthma and wheezing were also assessed using medical tests as well as questionnaires. The children's intake of both whole grains and fish was significantly linked to the incidence of wheezing and current asthma. They came to the conclusion that increasing consumption of whole grains could reduce the risk of childhood asthma by about 50 per cent.

OREGANO

Oregano herb is widely known as a potent germ-killer, anti-inflammatory and pain reliever. It is also being widely studied within the scientific community for its vast medical uses.

In research done on its volatile oil, it has been found that it could supersede many commonly-used pain killers, such as aspirin and even morphine with the added benefit that it is has little to zero side effects. Oregano has extremely high levels of free radical-fighting antioxidants, agents that protect the body from the development of chronic conditions over time.

FROM THE LABS

A study from the US Department of Agriculture showed that oregano essential oils presented antimicrobial activities against Salmonella and E. coli. Studies from the Department of Food Science at the University of Tennessee and the University of the Algarve found similar results for oregano's anti-bacterial action on pathogenic germs.

A recent study from the Department of Physiology and Biophysics at Georgetown University Medical Center, stated the following in regard to its use for preventing infections:

"New, safe, anti-microbial agents are needed to prevent and overcome severe bacterial, viral, and fungal infections. Based on our previous experience and that of others, we postulated that herbal essential oils, such as those of Origanum (oregano oil) offer such possibilities."

PEANUTS

Peanuts belong to the legume family of beans and lentils. Peanut pods grow underground and have a shell exterior with two or more peanut beans. Raw peanuts are high in several vitamins and minerals, and provide many proven health benefits.

FROM THE LABS

The antioxidants and folic acid in peanuts may provide some protection against cancer. A study in Taiwan found that eating peanuts reduced the chance of colo-rectal cancer by 27 per cent in men and 58 per cent in women.

Raw peanuts protect the gall bladder and assist in correcting fat metabolism. People who consume at least an ounce of peanuts each week reduce their chance of developing gall stones by 25 per cent.

The high monounsaturated fats in peanuts are good for your heart and could reduce the risk of cardiovascular disease by lowering LDL ('bad') cholesterol. The vitamin E content in these nuts benefits the skin, moisturizes the body, and keeps hair healthy. This vitamin is also shown to be excellent for the heart and brain.

PRAWNS/SHRIMP

While shrimp may be small, they are huge in their appeal as these deliciously clean and crisp tasting crustaceans can be served hot or cold, and are the most popular seafood in the world, next to fish. The firm, translucent, flesh of raw shrimp is low in saturated fat making it a healthier alternative to meat proteins. Fresh and frozen shrimp is available throughout the year.

FROM THE LABS

Shrimp is an excellent source of selenium; this neutralizes the injurious effects of free radicals which is the main cause of degenerative diseases.

It is a very good source of vitamin D required to regulate the absorption of calcium and phosphorus, which is essential for strong teeth and bones. It is a good source of vitamin B12, a vitamin that plays an important role for the proper brain function and essential for the formation and maturation of blood cells.

Prawns are also a good source of omega-3 fatty acids which reduce the risk of cardiovascular problems because it reduces cholesterol in the blood. Omega-3 fatty acids can also ease the symptoms of premenstrual syndrome, avoid blood clots, prevent the development of rheumatoid arthritis, slows the growth of cancerous tumours, and helps prevent Alzheimer's disease, besides having anti-inflammatory qualities.

RED LENTILS

These lentils are a type of pulse with lens-shaped seeds. Red lentils have the most distinctive flavour and are most easily cooked of all lentils. Many nutritionists recommend lentils as an excellent source of proteins, especially to vegetarians and vegans. Lentils are known to fill the iron stores in your body, are a great source of dietary fibres, help in stabilizing blood sugar levels, and provide a constant and steady energy to your body. Lentils provide important minerals and vitamins (folate and thiamine). They contain molybdenum, manganese, iron, phosphorus, copper and potassium.

FROM THE LABS

Legume family to which red lentils belong is proven to be connected to the significant decrease of heart problem; it has been estimated that the risks are decreased by nearly 82 per cent and the fibres, folate (vitamin B6), and magnesium present in lentils is responsible for this heart related effect.

SESAME

Small is big. Those unfamiliar with sesame seeds are surprised that such a tiny, flat seed, only 1/8 inch in length and 1/20 of an inch thick, can be endowed with such depth of flavour. In its raw form, it is frequently described as delicately sweet and nutty with an earthy bouquet. Sesame seeds are 25 per cent protein and are especially rich in methionine and tryptophan (amino acids), often lacking in adequate quantities in many plant proteins. One ounce of decorticated or hulled seeds contains 6 grams of protein, 3.7 grams of fibre and 14 grams of total fat. When toasted they lose all their nutrients. The fat in sesame seeds is 38% per cent monounsaturated, and 44% polyunsaturated which equals 82% unsaturated fatty acids. There is often concern that vegans do not get a sufficient amount of zinc in their diet. Include sesame tahini (a paste made by grounding sesame seeds) in your diet often and reap the benefit of plenty of zinc with one tablespoon supplying 1.17 mg. Both natural and hulled sesame seeds contain healthy amounts of the B vitamins riboflavin, thiamine, and niacin. With natural seeds scoring 8.7 mcg of folic acid for 1 tablespoon and plenty of vitamin B6, you can count on sesame seeds for excellent nourishment.

> ### Interesting!!
> Early Assyrians believed their Gods drank sesame wine as a prelude to creating the world.

SUNFLOWER SEEDS

They are more commonly eaten as a healthy snack than as a part of a meal. The seeds may be sold as in-shell seeds or de-hulled kernels. They can also be sprouted and eaten in salads. De-hulling is commonly performed by cracking the hull with one's teeth and spitting it out while keeping the kernel in the mouth and eating it.

FROM THE LABS

Sunflower seeds are a powerhouse of nutrients. It is rich in vitamin E, thiamine, manganese, magnesium, copper, selenium, phosphorus and folate. They are one of the richest sources of vitamin E. By obstructing oxidation of cholesterol, vitamin E prevents formation of plagues on the walls of our cardiac blood vessels. Magnesium is one of the minerals that can normalize the blood pressure level and sunflower seeds are a good source of magnesium.

They contain selenium. Studies have found that selenium could be effective in preventing the growth of malignant cells. Selenium is needed to accelerate the repair of damaged DNA. It also helps the cell to manufacture DNA. It obstructs development of cancer cells and encourages the body to remove abnormal cells.

> ### Interesting!!
> In Turkey and Israel, sunflower seeds can be bought as a common stadium food eaten while watching sports.

WALNUTS

From ancient times through the nineteenth century herbalists prescribed the walnut, the bark, the roots, and the leaves as an astringent, a laxative, a purgative to induce vomiting, a styptic to stop bleeding, a vermifuge to expel worms or parasites, and a hepatic to tone the liver. The walnut served to induce sweating, cure diarrhoea, soothe sore gums and skin diseases, cure herpes, and relieve inflamed tonsils.

WALNUTS REPRESENT LONGEVITY

In one region of southern France known as Perigord, the long-standing traditional diet is very high in fried foods, rich meats, and fatty patés. Yet, the people suffer fewer heart attacks than their counterparts in other countries. At first, medical experts explained this phenomenon by attributing this miracle to the red wine they drink. Yet, the residents of this region didn't drink any more red wine than those in other parts of Europe. Closer examination revealed that their daily green salads were dressed with walnut oil and chopped walnuts, helping to lower their levels of LDL and overall cholesterol in the blood stream.

A study published in the American Journal of Clinical Nutrition, May 1994, showed that those whose diets included nuts, either walnuts or almonds, were able to lower their LDL cholesterol by 9 to 10% per cent.

INCREASED RESISTANCE POWER

The nut itself has been used to prevent weight gain, calm hysteria, eliminate morning sickness, and to strengthen one's constitution. Walnuts are rich in protein, providing 7 grams for that same one-fourth cup, 2 grams of fibre, and only 7 grams of carbohydrates. Walnuts can be considered a super food because they contain a full complement of vitamins, including B1, B2, B3, B5, B6 and folic acid. They also contain a wealth of minerals, such as iron, magnesium, potassium and zinc.

Walnuts contain vitamin E – alpha, beta, delta and gamma-tocopherol, making it exceptionally high in antioxidants.

Interesting!!

There is a legend that presumes walnuts were one of the gifts presented to Jesus by the three wise men.

WHOLE WHEAT

Making a commitment to eat whole grains is an advanced healthy diet technique that has a lot in common with eating only organic produce. This commitment will add quality to your children's diet and is well worth the health benefits they will derive.

FROM THE LABS

Results of an extensive study conducted on whole grains concluded that "Most whole-grain wheat kernels are composed of 80% per cent endosperm (the predominant component of refined flour, which is rich in starch and protein but poor in most micronutrients), 15% per cent bran (a major source of fibre, micronutrients, antioxidants, and phytochemicals), and 5% per cent germ (plant embryo). However, refined grain products and their fibre do not appear to confer health-protective effects; this suggests that these health benefits do not lie in the endosperm. Furthermore, this same study strongly pointed out that the grain's bran component may contain the most important bioactive constituents."

Interesting!!

The Roman goddess, Ceres, who was deemed protector of the grain, gave grains their common name today–"Cereal."

TOOLS FOR IMMUNITY BUILDING

Many people are under the false impression that delicious healthy food making demands a degree in cuisine, a chef's hat, and a big time commitment. This is absolutely not true. And the proof of that is given in the recipes below. They have been created to be exceptionally flavourful and with the express goal of making healthy eating even quicker and easier than the typical breakfast or lunch you are preparing even now. Once you adapt to this way of meal making, you will find that it even transfers readily to your favourite recipes, improving their nutritional quality and cutting down their preparation time.

WELLNESS FOOD APPEALS TO ALL OUR SENSES

When parents think of healthy eating, they often assume they will have to sacrifice taste and the enjoyment of their children's food. However, nothing could be farther from the truth. Part of the beauty of rejuvenative foods is the inherent freshness that they emanate, a vitality that comes across in their rich and lively flavour. The vibrant taste of these foods is one of the major reasons that people across the globe are using more and more of these healthy food ingredients in the meals they prepare. Just imagining the smooth creamy taste of a melon, the musky sweet flavour of a ripe mango, or the nutty chewiness of almonds, or even the fresh crispness of cabbage leaves is sure to please the palates of both the very young and the teens.

All recipes used for **'the 12 week incredible immunity plan'** are:

1. Quick to prepare - less than 35 minutes
2. Made with familiar ingredients
3. Clear and easy to understand
4. Affordable
5. Made from ingredients available most of the year
6. Good tasting
7. Healthy and nutritious besides having the ability to give you magical results within 12 weeks!!

LIQUID GOLD

EMERGE REGENERATED

INGREDIENTS

1. 8 dates, brown or black
2. 3 green cardamoms
3. 1 tsp fennel seeds
4. 4-5 white pepper corns
5. 300 ml purified water
6. 2 tsp crushed ice

Quick, easy and delicious! This date smoothie recipe comes from many years of enjoying Middle East cuisine. They like to sneak in a hearty drink before breakfast. Your children will grow to love it.

GETTING READY

1. Wash dates, de-seed them and soak them for 8 hours along with fennel seeds and cardamoms in 300 ml water.
2. Crush the white pepper corns into a fine powder.

LET'S START

1. Put soaked dates in the blender along with other ingredients. Do not discard the soaking water.
2. Blend them well, gradually adding the water in which they were soaked.
3. Add white pepper powder.
4. Strain and chill or serve at room temperature.
5. Drink immediately.

NOTE

Quantity of dates can depend on the variety or the quality of dates you use, since sweetness of dates can vary with the quality.

ENERGY BOOSTER

INGREDIENTS

1. 4 black pepper corns
2. 5 prunes
3. ½ vanilla bean, dried Or ¼ tsp natural vanilla essence
4. 250 ml purified water

The recipe for this smoothie is our family is favourite. It's easy to prepare and perfect for the quick send off children require in the morning. We make this with natural vanilla giving it a lovely appetizing aroma.

GETTING READY

1. Chop and crush vanilla bean.
2. Soak prunes, crushed vanilla bean with the black pepper corns for 8 hours in purified water.
3. Put vanilla essence in water if that is your choice.

LET'S START

1. Strain water in container and keep aside.
2. Blend the fleshy prunes, vanilla bean and pepper corns.
3. Add soaking water gradually, into the blender to allow it to turn into a smooth and silky drink.
4. Keep it to cool in refrigerator or serve immediately to energize your child for the entire day.

FUEL FOR BEAUTY

INGREDIENTS

1. 1 stone fruit, medium sized, ripe and yellow
2. 1 tsp honey
3. 1 green cardamom,
4. 4 black pepper corns
5. Purified water

This is a great summer drink. Refreshing to the throat and soothing to the stomach. Stone apple is known to remove all toxic waste from the intestine including worms, if any. Tasty and therapeutic!

GETTING READY

1. Grind green cardamom and black pepper corns.
2. Crack bael fruit into two halves.
3. Scoop out all the flesh in a bowl.

LET'S START

1. Add some water to the flesh and mash into a pulp. Strain well through strainer to remove the seeds and all the fibre.
2. As the juice trickles down into the bowl, add some more water to the juice so as to make the consistency of the juice to your liking.
3. Pour it in your glass stirring in honey, powdered green cardamom and pepper corns.
4. Serve cold.

LET 'ER' RIP

INGREDIENTS

1. 2 red apples, large, hard & juicy
2. 3 – 4 figs
3. 20 basil leaves, fresh
4. 4 black pepper corns
5. 100 ml purified water

A perfect start for the day. Sweet and nutritious – this mixture of apples with figs is excellent for growing kids with its rich calcium and iron content.

GETTING READY

1. Wash and soak figs overnight in 100 ml water. You will be using this fig water to prepare the smoothie.
2. Wash and scrub apples to remove the wax layer on the peel. Core them.

LET'S START

1. Put soaked figs, basil leaves and peppercorns in a blender. Churn while adding fig-soaked water until it becomes creamy in consistency.
2. Add remaining water and churn again. Remove and keep in deep freezer to chill.
3. Slice the apples without peeling them. Juice them in the juicer.
4. Mix apple juice with the chilled, blended figs in the blender.
5. Pour in a glass to serve.

Bunches of fresh basil may be frozen and stored successfully for a few weeks. The best method is to place a small bunch in a clean plastic supermarket bag, blow some air in to inflate it, and place in the freezer where it will not be squashed. You will find it quite convenient to then nip off just a few of these frozen leaves when they are required.

REVITALIZER

INGREDIENTS

1. 2 bananas, ripe with brown flecks
2. 1 coconut, fresh
3. 2 pods green cardamom
4. 1 tsp honey
5. water from the coconut
6. 100 ml plain water
7. 2 tsp crushed ice (optional)

We have used bananas and sometimes we put in fresh mangoes or chikoos and a dash of cinnamon. It turns out wonderful and gives seasonal nutrients for your loved ones.

GETTING READY

1. Choose ripe bananas and remove their peel.
2. Crush the green cardamoms into powder.
3. Prepare coconut milk with 100 ml water, in addition to its own water as described in a separate section.

LET'S START

1. Chop bananas into chunks and put them in the blender.
2. Add crushed green cardamom and honey. Blend to a creamy consistency.
3. Add prepared coconut milk and churn once to mix well. Pour into a glass and top with crushed ice if your child likes cold drinks.
4. Your child will love its heavenly taste!

Experiments conducted on honey show that its bactericide properties increase twofold when diluted with water. This bactericide (bacteria-killing) property of honey is named "the inhibition effect". It is very interesting to note that newly born bees in the colony are nourished with diluted honey by the bees responsible for their supervision - as if they know this feature of the honey.

RIDE'EM HIGH

INGREDIENTS

1. 2 mangoes, ripe and sweet, non-fibrous variety
2. 35 almonds
3. ¼ Thai ginger root, fresh
4. ½ tsp honey
5. pinch of cinnamon
6. 200 ml water
7. 4 tsp crushed ice (optional)

Qualifying for the tag of mega nutrition, this delectable milk shake will allow your child to enjoy mango throughout the year. Great brain booster and growth enhancer.

GETTING READY

1. Prepare almond milk as given in a separate section.
2. Wash, peel and cut mangoes into large chunks. Freeze them until you prepare almond milk.
3. Scrape ginger, wash and cut it.

LET'S START

1. Blend ginger with almond milk. Add cinnamon powder to flavour the milk.
2. Immediately add chilled chunks of mangoes to almond milk. Churn until smooth in consistency.
3. Stir in honey.
4. Pour in a tall glass and top it with crushed ice.
5. Serve this delicious mango almond smoothie immediately.

NOTE

You can freeze mango chunks when the fruit is in season and use it whenever you require. This type of home freezing is better than using chemical controlled preservation done in fruits available in the market.

VEGGIE MAGIC

INGREDIENTS

1. 250 ml coconut milk, freshly prepared
2. 1 red bell pepper, small
3. $1/4$ ginger root, fresh
4. 4 pods garlic
5. $1/3$ tsp black pepper corns
6. few sprigs coriander leaves, fresh
7. 10 curry leaves, fresh
8. 20 mint leaves, fresh
9. Rock salt to taste

This is the only way many mothers have convinced their children to drink 'milk'. Fresh coconut milk is rich in protein, calcium and minerals. The fatty acids are an added bonus for the brain. 60 per cent of the brain is made of fats making it your body's fattest organ.

GETTING READY

1. Wash bell pepper, rubbing in the crevices to remove all dirt. Cut in half and remove seeds.
2. Peel and wash ginger.
3. Remove covering from the garlic pods.
4. Wash all the green leaves thoroughly under running tap water.
5. Prepare coconut milk as described in a separate section, 250 ml in quantity and chill it. Grind the black pepper corns.

LET'S START

1. Chop the bell pepper into chunks and finely shred the green leaves.
2. Put the above chunks, garlic, ginger and the chopped green leaves into the blender. Churn to make a smooth paste.
3. Start adding the fresh coconut milk and gradually blend all of it.
4. Stir in the salt and black pepper.
5. Ask your child to sip it slowly and enjoy the real nutri-milk.

2 FRUIT MÉLANGES

BOUNDLESS ENERGY

INGREDIENTS

1. 3 bananas, large and ripe
2. ½ pineapple or 4 thick round slices, fresh
3. 1 pear
4. 1 kiwi
5. 5 walnuts, whole

Toss this fruit breakfast together in minutes. Made with sweet bananas, tangy pineapple and tossed walnuts, the flavours in this meal go together wonderfully, and create a beautiful looking fruit medley.

GETTING READY

1. Choose fully ripened bananas with brown flecks. The potent quality of this meal is dependent on the natural sugar in them.
2. Soak walnuts overnight. Remove their skin.
3. Prepare the pineapple by peeling; core it and removing the eyes.
4. Wash and scrub the pear.

LET'S START

1. Slice the pineapple and then extract juice from 3 thick slices.
2. Cut one banana into chunks and put in the blender. Pour pineapple juice over it and churn mixing the two well. Keep this pineapple sauce separately.

3. Chop pear, kiwi, one slice of pineapple and the remaining two bananas.
4. Add the cut fruit to the bowl.
5. Pour the pineapple-banana sauce over the fruit evenly.
6. Chop the peeled walnuts and garnish the fruit bowl with walnuts.
7. Refrigerate for 15 minutes before serving.

> *Kiwi fruits are so delicious that they can be eaten as it is. They can be peeled with a paring knife and then sliced or you can cut them in half and scoop the flesh out with a spoon. Children can also enjoy the skin which is very thin like pears and is full of nutrients and fibre; the peach-like fuzz can be rubbed off before eating.*

CELEBRATE CHILDHOOD

INGREDIENTS

1. 1 melon of your choice, large and aromatic
2. ½ ginger root, fresh
3. 20 leaves of mint, fresh
4. 1 green cardamom
5. 1 tsp organic honey
6. Crushed ice

Super simple! Cantaloupe, honey dew or musk melon, choose your child's favourite and add the spice and herbs. A dollop of honey makes it a fantastic tongue pleaser.

GETTING READY

1. Choose a sweet and ripe melon with a strong aroma. Wash well and peel it.
2. Coarsely crush seeds of green cardamom.
3. Wash ginger & mint leaves. Peel the ginger root.

LET'S START

1. Chop ginger and mint leaves. Put them in the blender along with the crushed cardamom.
2. Add two 2" thick slices of melon, chopped.
3. Put honey in it and churn the blender to make a smooth cream of melon and other ingredients.
4. Slice and chop the remaining melon into 1" cubes and keep in fruit bowl. Pour the blended melon cream over the chopped fruit.
5. Garnish with few leaves of chopped mint.
6. Chill if serving on a holiday or place in tiffin box. As your loved ones partake this meal, their body's cells celebrate rejuvenation.

Fruit Mélanges

COLOURS OF HEALTH

INGREDIENTS

1. 500 gm papaya, ripe and orange-yellow in colour
2. 1 apple, large
3. 1 kiwi, ripe and firm
4. 1 pomegranate, kandhari preferable (deep red variety)
5. 4 walnuts, whole or 8 halves

This mélange of fresh fruits is so colourful; it nearly pulls the kids to eat it. Intrigued with yellow, white, green and ruby red; children learn how health comes from a rainbow of colours.

GETTING READY

1. Soak walnuts overnight. Remove skin and chop them at the time of preparing this exotic meal.
2. Peel and de-seed the papaya.
3. Remove the outer covering from the pomegranate.
4. Wash apple thoroughly, scraping it under running water without scathing its skin.

LET'S START

1. Dice papaya into clean cubes and take out pomegranate seeds.
2. Wash and cut kiwi with its peel. Core out the seeds of the apple. Chop both apple and kiwi into clean, small cubes.
3. Put pomegranate seeds in the blender with 4 walnuts (halves) and blend into smooth consistency.
4. Toss all chopped and cubed fruit in a bowl and pour the creamy pomegranate sauce over the fruit.
5. Top them with pieces of remaining walnut after placing in school lunch box. Children really relish this 'Colours of Health'.

> Kiwi fruits should not be kept too long after cutting since they contain enzymes that act as a food tenderizer, with the ability to further tenderize the kiwi fruit itself and make it overly soft. Consequently, if you are adding kiwi fruit to fruit salad, you should do so at the last minute so as to prevent the other fruits from becoming too soggy.

FORTUNE FOR VITALS

INGREDIENTS

1. 2 red apples, medium
2. 1 pomegranate, small
3. 2 pears, medium
4. 2 oranges
5. Few sprigs of mint, fresh
6. Pinch of cinnamon powder

Sweeten your children's morning with this nifty way to prepare fruits and spices. Rich in antioxidants and natural sugars, this mixture invigorates the whole body.

GETTING READY

1. Grind cinnamon to make fresh powder for best aroma and potency.
2. Apply lemon juice on the chopping board to prevent apples and pears from turning brown. Wash and core pears.
3. Peel pomegranate and neatly take out the pomegranate kernels.
4. Wash and scrape apples to use the skin of the fruit.

LET'S START

1. Juice oranges and pour the juice in the bowl. Grind ¼ of pomegranate seeds.
2. Core the apples and cut into small cubes. Immediately drop them in the bowl to soak them in orange juice
3. Cut pears in small cubes. Drop them in the bowl of orange juice.
4. Mix in ground creamy pomegranate seeds to the fruit.
5. Stir in powdered cinnamon. Sprinkle rest of the pomegranate on top.
6. Garnish with refreshing mint sprigs before serving.

Fruit is pre-digested and biologically accepted by a human body. Eating fruit in the right combinations is the important key to benefit from them, otherwise it tends to make the body hyperacidic.

Fruit Mélanges

MORNING MANTRA

INGREDIENTS

1. 4 bananas, large and ripe with brown flecks
2. 2 oranges
3. 2 apples
4. 15 almonds, mamara variety preferable
5. 10 strawberries (Optional)

A big change from the usual rotis and vegetables for tiffin, this fruit and nut combination offers the best of seasonal fruits and the year round ones. An excellent option, different from the everyday fare.

GETTING READY

1. Buy bananas 3 days prior to using them. They need to be completely ripe with brown dots or flecks, so wrap them in newspaper to convert the starch into sugar. Check every day for readiness.
2. Soak almonds overnight.

LET'S START

1. Peel almonds, cut into julienne shape and keep them aside.
2. Peel and chop 3 bananas into cubes. Put fourth banana in the blender.
3. Peel oranges, de-seed and remove the white part from them. Take half and put in the bowl with the cubed bananas and the remaining half into the blender.
4. Wash and chop apple into small cubes. Add them to the bowl of bananas and oranges.
5. Wash and chop strawberries. Put half in the blender and add the rest to the almonds.
6. Blend the fruit in the blender to creamy consistency.

7. Pour this cream in the bowl of chopped fruit and mix all together.
8. Garnish with almonds and strawberries.
9. Chill if you want before serving this delightful breakfast.

> Whenever using apples in any recipe, take a knife and gently scrape the sides of the fruit. You will be surprised to see a layer of wax coming off it. This wax is usually put to preserve the freshness of the fruit, or to prevent insects from attacking it. Always scrape the peel right before using it or else the colour of the apple from outside can change and it will look unpalatable.

3 PLATE OF PANACEA

CHINESE TOSSED VEGGIES

INGREDIENTS

1. 200 gm broccoli, small head
2. 1 carrot, Medium
3. 1 red bell pepper
4. 1 green bell pepper
5. 1 yellow bell pepper
6. 4 spring onions
7. 1 ginger root, fresh
8. 6 garlic pods
9. 2 tsp soy sauce
10. 1 tsp Lemon juice
11. 1 tsp extra virgin olive oil
12. Salt to taste

A welcome addition to your range of breakfast for your children. Every child we know loves chowmein and this recipe is made exactly the same way minus the noodles.

GETTING READY

1. Cut Broccoli into small florets and soak them in salt warm water for 20 minutes.
2. Mince ginger and garlic. Slice spring onions and chop them. Cut its green stalk into juliennes.
3. Cut bell peppers into 1 cm squares.
4. Peel and scoop-out the eyes of the carrot. Wash and chop into juliennes.

LET'S START

1. Heat pan and pour oil. At the same time add minced ginger, garlic paste and chopped onion. Stir them for a while.
2. Add julienned carrot and stir for a while again.
3. Add broccoli and green pepper. Cook for a while and add soy sauce, green of onion, bell peppers and salt and stir them.
4. Cover the pan and cook the vegetable retaining their crunchiness. Transfer the vegetables from the pan to the bowl. Squeeze lemon juice and toss them.
5. Serve hot or transfer to school lunch box.
6. Keep some lemon wedges on the side.

FEAST TODAY

INGREDIENTS

1. 1 cup brown chick peas, dried
2. ½ cup green peas, dried
3. 4 baby corns
4. 1 red bell pepper
5. 1" ginger root, fresh
6. 10 almonds
7. 1 tsp tahini
8. 2 indian gooseberries
9. 1 tsp lemon juice
10. 1 tsp extra virgin olive oil
11. Salt to taste

If your child is a gusto eater, then he would love the earthy taste of this wholesome breakfast. Rich with nuts and seeds, you can be rest assured he has got the best nourishment in the morning.

GETTING READY

1. Soak dehydrated green peas for 6 hours. Drain water. Allow them to sprout for the next 2-3 days.
2. Soak chick peas and almonds separately overnight.
3. Chop baby corns.
4. Wash bell pepper and de-seed it. Chop half of the bell pepper.
5. Wash and grate indian gooseberries.

LET'S START

1. Drain water of chick peas and steam them in minimum water. Put them in a bowl and sprinkle salt.
2. Wash green pea's sprouts. Drain water well. Sauté sprouts in olive oil for 3 minutes.
3. Turn them out in the bowl. Add to the bowl chopped baby corn, bell pepper and grated indian gooseberries.
4. Grind ½ bell pepper along with ginger and lemon juice. Pour blended lemony bell pepper.
5. Toss all ingredients.
6. Serve.

ROBUST TRANSITION

INGREDIENTS

1. 1 cup sweet corn
2. 50 gm parsley or corainder leaves, fresh
3. 2 onions, Small
4. 1 red bell-pepper
5. 1 cucumber
6. ½ tsp extra virgin olive oil
7. Lemon juice to taste
8. Black salt to taste

Zesty and mouth watering! Make it spicy by adding a green chilli and you have a sure winner on your hands. Even the fussiest of kids ask for it again and again.

GETTING READY

1. Soak parsley/coriander in salt water for 30 minutes. Rinse parsley in plain water.
2. Wash red bell pepper, de-seed and chop finely.
3. Peel onions and cut in round rings.
4. Remove corn from the cob.
5. Peel cucumber and chop it finely.

LET'S START

1. Sauté corn kernels in a non-stick pan using olive oil. Keep pan covered while cooking. Once corn kernels become tender, transfer them to a bowl.
2. Add chopped onion, bell pepper and cucumber into the bowl.
3. Put parsley and lemon juice in a blender and blend coarsely. Add to bowl and mix all the ingredients.
4. Sprinkle salt and toss.
5. Serve at room temperature

TASTY TANGLES

INGREDIENTS

1. 50 gm vermicelli
2. 200 gm cauliflower
3. 2 onions
4. 2 tomatoes, red and ripe
5. ½ ginger root, fresh
6. ½ cinnamon stick
7. 2 garlic pods
8. Few sprigs of coriander leaves, fresh
9. 1 tsp extra virgin olive oil
10. Salt and pepper to taste

This very flavourful dish is easy to prepare. It has a nice texture and the aroma is inviting…..A nice hearty breakfast that nourishes supremely.

GETTING READY

1. Cut cauliflower florets and soak in salt water. Peel and slice onions.
2. Chop coriander leaves.
3. Crush garlic and ginger.
4. Wash and blanch tomatoes. Remove its skin and add salt and puree.
5. Grind cinnamon stick to powder.

LET'S START

1. Boil water. Cut vermicelli into 1" length and put in boiling water. Put off flame.
2. Leave vermicelli in water till it turns transparent and soft. Strain and transfer them into cold water. Leave for a while. Drain and keep aside.
3. Heat a non-stick pan. Add oil, onion, garlic and ginger. Stir and cook for a while.
4. Add cauliflower to the pan. Cover the pan and cook till cauliflower is tender.
5. Add vermicelli to the pan and mix with cauliflower.
6. Add puree of tomato and toss vermicelli and cauliflower. Put off the flame.
7. Sprinkle cinnamon powder. Keep the pan covered for a while.
8. Garnish with coriander leaves before serving.

SOUTHERN DELICACY

INGREDIENTS

1. 1 cup semolina
2. 150 gm green peas, fresh and unshelled
3. Few fenugreek leaves, fresh or 1 tsp dried fenugreek
4. 1 green chilli
5. 1 lemon
6. 1 tsp eno salt
7. ½ tsp black mustard seeds
8. Salt to taste

Basically a south Indian steamed recipe and a great filling breakfast which can be varied for wholesome nutritional contents.

GETTING READY

1. Shell peas, wash them and coarsely grind them.
2. Wash fenugreek leaves and cut them very finely.
3. Cut green chilli very finely.
4. Roast semolina for 2-3 minutes. Cool it and pack it in a jar to make it ready for use.

LET'S START

1. Mix roasted semolina, peas, chopped fenugreek leaves, green chillies and salt. Beat well and add little water to make a smooth batter.
2. Mix well so that there is no lump left in the batter. Leave it for 15-20 minutes.
3. Add eno salt and mix again. Grease idli moulds and pour batter in each mould.
4. Place the idli moulds in a pressure cooker. Steam for 12-15 minutes.
6. Heat oil in a pan and splutter mustard seeds on it. Add sliced green chillies as well.
7. Pour on idlis as they are taken out of the steamer.
8. Serve with coconut chutney.

BRILLIANCE CRAFT

INGREDIENTS

1. ½ cup whole wheat flour
2. ½ cup semolina
3. 1 cup sprouted mung beans
4. 1 onion
5. ½ ginger root, fresh
6. 2 garlic pods
7. 1 green chili
8. Few mint leaves, fresh
9. Salt to taste
10. Water as required

The answer to every mom's prayer for the perfect tiffin! Filled with protein rich mung beans, these paranthas taste extraordinary with curd blends or sauces of choice.

GETTING READY

1. Soak mung beans for 8 hours. Drain water and tie in a muslin cloth.
2. Keep beans in a warm place for 12 hours. Wash them and again keep them covered at a warm place for 8 hours.
3. Keep sprouted mung beans in the refrigerator. They will keep for a week. Wash sprouts before using.
4. Peel and chop onion, ginger and garlic very finely. Wash mint leaves.

LET'S START

1. Put sprouted pulse, green chilli and mint leaves in a blender. Blend them coarsely.
2. Turn over blended pulse and chopped onion etc. in dough-maker utensil.
3. Add salt and wheat flour and mix them well with hand.
4. Now, add water gradually to make a dough and make equal size round balls.
5. Using a rolling pin, make thin round shapes and cook on a non-stick griddle. Apply extra virgin olive oil.
6. Relish them with raita or a chutney of your choice.

WALNUTTY SANDWICHES

Filled with greens and nuts, these meal in hand sandwiches are great to munch on during the lunch break in school. The multigrain bread rounds off the nutrient content.

INGREDIENTS

1. 4 whole grain or multigrain bread slices
2. 5 walnuts, whole or 10 halves
3. 5 leaves iceberg lettuce
4. 1 onion, small
5. 1 green chilli
6. 10 mint leaves, fresh
7. 1 tsp hung curd
8. Black salt to taste
9. White pepper to taste

GETTING READY

1. Soak walnuts overnight. Peel them in the morning.
2. Wash iceberg leaves and soak them in salt water
3. Peel and chop onion finely.
4. Wash and chop very finely mint leaves, nuts and green chilli.

LET'S START

1. Combine chopped onion, nuts, green chilli and mint in a bowl.
2. Add hung curd, salt and white pepper. This is the filling between the two toasts.
3. Grill toasts.
4. Place iceberg leaves on the toasts and place the filling between the two toasts.
5. Slice them into two rectangular halves and serve.

NOTE

Do not cook or heat while filling is inside otherwise the curd will curdle.

TURBO CHARGER

INGREDIENTS

1. 1 cup moth beans sprouts
2. ½ cup red lentil sprout
3. 1 tomato, red and ripe
4. 1 onion
5. 1 red or 1 yellow bell pepper
6. 1 carrot, small
7. 2 garlic pods
8. 1 green chilli
9. Few coriander leaves, fresh
10. 2 tsp sunflower seeds
11. Lemon juice to taste
12. 1 tsp extra virgin olive oil
13. Salt to taste

During our test kitchen stage, this breakfast was the most asked for by children. Later we got to know that kids taking it to school had to carry extra portions for their classmates.

GETTING READY

1. Soak sunflower seeds for 2 hours. Drain water and keep aside.
2. Wash and drain sprouts.
3. Mince garlic, green chillies and carrot.
4. Peel and chop onion finely.
5. Wash and chop bell pepper and tomato.

LET'S START

1. Stir-fry the chopped bell pepper, tomato along with onion for about 1 minute.
2. Add minced carrot, garlic and green chilli to the above vegetables in the pan.
3. Cover the pan and put off the flame. Keep the pan covered for 5 minutes.
4. Separately sauté sprouts without adding any water, retaining their natural crunchiness and yet becoming tender.
5. Add steamed sprouts to the pan and sprinkle salt and lemon juice. Toss all ingredients to mix well.
6. Mix finely chopped coriander leaves and sprinkle sunflower seeds on top.
7. Enjoy this mega rich micronutrient meal at school or at home.

TEMPTED

The taste of street food is loved by all. An Indian street food speciality that becomes an instant favourite of kids anywhere in the world. Delightful and scrumptious!

INGREDIENTS

1. 250 gm white peas, dried
2. 1 onion
3. 1 tomato, red and ripe
4. 1 cucumber, small
5. 1 green chilli
6. 1" ginger root, fresh
7. 1 tsp cumin seeds, roasted and ground
8. 1 tsp coriander seed powder
9. Lemon juice to taste
10. Black salt to taste

GETTING READY

1. Soak white peas for 6-7 hours.
2. Wash and chop finely green chillies and tomato.
3. Peel and chop onion and cucumber.
4. Wash ginger rhizome and chop in juliennes.

LET'S START

1. Pressure cook white peas in minimum water and salt to taste. Steam for one whistle or till tender. Avoid adding any soda bicarbonate while cooking.
2. Put steamed peas in a large bowl along with any cooking water left.
3. Add chopped vegetables.
4. Squeeze lemon juice.
5. Sprinkle cumin, coriander powder, black salt and toss.
6. Garnish with julienned ginger before serving.

MASTER YOUR METABOLISM

INGREDIENTS

1. 1 cup semolina
2. 1 onion
3. 1 green capsicum
4. 4 garlic pods
5. 1" ginger root, fresh
6. 1 green chilli
7. Few curry leaves, fresh
8. 1 lemon
9. ¼ tsp baking powder
10. 1 cup water

Forget about bland or mild! This South Indian treat- 'uttapam' or pancakes made with veggies, go lip smackingly with a robust coconut sauce.

GETTING READY

1. Make a smooth and thick batter of semolina with water.
2. Crush ginger and garlic to take out juice.
3. Add baking powder and juice of ginger and garlic to the semolina batter. Mix well.
4. Add lemon juice and mix again.

LET'S START

1. Spread semolina batter on a griddle. Cook on low flame.
2. Sprinkle chopped onion and green capsicum along with curry leaves on top. Cover the griddle and cook for a minute.
3. Turn the side upside down and cook for another minute.
4. Serve with coconut chutney from **'Mixed Bag section'**.

4 THE SALAD POT

Salads are the fast food for a healthy nation. They are easy and simple to make. You only have to cut, chop and mix. There is no cooking time involved and neither the devitalisation of nutrients due to high heat.

RAW PAW SALAD

Toothsome! Raw papaya has hundreds of benefits and is widely used in Indian, Thai and Malaysian cuisines. We learnt to use this super food especially for children.

INGREDIENTS

1. 1 raw papaya, small
2. 4 walnuts
3. 1 beetroot, small
4. 1 onion
5. few lettuce leaves (optional)
6. 1 tsp oregano, dried or few sprigs of oregano, fresh
7. 3 garlic pods
8. ½ tsp mustard powder
9. 2 tsp lemon juice
10. 1 tsp extra virgin olive oil
11. Black salt to taste

GETTING READY

1. Peel papaya and remove inner white skin properly.
2. De-eye beetroot, scrape gently and chop finely.
3. Wash lettuce leaves in salt water.
4. Cut onions into very thin long slices and separate them. Put in ice cold water for 5-10 minutes.

LET'S START

1. Layer the base of a salad bowl with lettuce leaves.
2. Grate papaya or chop very finely and put in a separate bowl.
3. Squeeze water and add onion to papaya.
4. Wash beetroot and chop it finely, mix in salt.
5. Crush garlic fine, squeeze lemon juice and mix both together.
6. Add olive oil, mustard powder and salt to lemon juice.
7. Mix this lemony mixture in the papaya bowl.
8. Spread this mixture on lettuce leaves in the salad bowl.
9. Top this salad with chopped beetroot.
10. Drizzle little lemon juice on it.
11. Chill for a while and serve with a meal.

THE BLOOD FIXER

Crunchy and crisp! The combination of veggies in this salad contains all the nutrients to clean the blood. An excellent skin nourisher from the inside out.

INGREDIENTS

1. 1 iceberg lettuce, full head
2. 1 carrot
3. ½ coconut, fresh
4. few coriander leaves, fresh
5. 1 green chilli
6. 1 tsp dry coriander seeds
7. 2 tsp curd
8. 6 almonds
9. black salt to taste

GETTING READY

1. Break open the coconut. Strain and keep its water aside. Scrape its brown skin and dice it.
2. De-eye the carrot, scrape it gently and then grate it.
3. Wash iceberg leaves in salt water and chop leaves.
4. Soak almonds overnight. Peel almonds and chop them.
5. Wash coriander leaves.

LET'S START

1. Grind coconut, coriander leaves, chilli and coriander seeds.
2. Add salt and curd.
3. Lace lettuce leaves with ground coconut sauce. Lay on a flat salad dish.
4. Add grated carrot, chopped iceberg lettuce and coriander leaves.
5. Top it with chopped almonds.

TRANSFORMATOR

When your child's hunger is low, give him this salad. It stimulates the stomach juices and whets up the appetite. Tangy yoghurt gets you the big thumbs up from your kid.

INGREDIENTS

1. 4 green cabbage leaves, large
2. 2 red cabbage leaves
3. 20 peanuts, raw
4. 1 yellow bell pepper, small
5. 3" coconut chunk, fresh
6. Few curry leaves, fresh and soft
7. 5 black pepper corns
8. 1 tsp hung curd
9. Salt to taste

GETTING READY

1. Soak peanuts overnight and remove their peel.
2. Wash green and red cabbage leaves rubbing their veins. Soak these leaves in salt water for 15-20 minutes.
3. Rinse and cut them into fine strips or thread-like juliennes.
4. Grind coconut and pepper corns coarsely.
5. Wash yellow pepper, remove seeds and chop.
6. Chop peanuts and curry leaves.

LET'S START

1. Place all the ingredients in a bowl.
2. Toss all ingredients along with curd and sprinkle salt.
3. Serve cool or at room temperature before serving the meal.

NATURAL BRAIN PROTECTOR

INGREDIENTS

1. 200 gm tofu
2. 2 carrots, medium
3. 1 yellow bell pepper
4. 100 gm green coriander leaves, fresh
5. ½ tsp yellow mustard seeds, ground
6. 1 lemon
7. Black salt to taste

The secret of anti-ageing of the Chinese – Tofu is the ace up your sleeve for getting your kids to eat and boost brain function. Homemade tofu literally melts in the mouth.

GETTING READY

1. Make fresh tofu according to recipe given in a separate section. Drain water to get scrambled tofu.
2. Wash, scrape and grate carrots.
3. Wash bell pepper well in the crevices. De-seed and chop it finely.
4. Wash and chop coriander leaves finely.

LET'S START

1. Put scrambled tofu, grated carrots and chopped bell pepper in a bowl.
2. Add ground mustard, salt and finely chopped coriander leaves.
3. Sprinkle lemon juice. Toss well by hand.
4. Keep this salad for 8-10 hrs at room temperature so as to release mustard flavour and taste.
5. Serve before meal at lunch.

FRESH 'N' JUICY

INGREDIENTS

1. 4 tomatoes, large, red and ripe
2. 2 spring onions
3. 20 green lettuce leaves
4. Few coriander leaves, fresh
5. 2 tsp lemon juice
6. 4 garlic pods
7. ½" ginger root, fresh
8. 3 black pepper corns
9. Black salt to taste

NOTE
Raw tomatoes and cooked cereals like roti or rice make an acidic combination. It is best to get the antioxidant lycopene from raw tomatoes in a meal composed of vegetables of your choice, dals or chicken without rotis and breads.

Peppery and piquant! It is the conversion of the simple home salad into a delicacy. You can always substitute the coriander leaves with herbs of choice. Try oregano, mint, and thyme for starters.

GETTING READY

1. Wash all the vegetables.
2. Shred the green lettuce.
3. Chop ginger, garlic and coriander leaves.
4. Cut spring onions along with their greens into juliennes.
5. Make wedges of tomatoes.

LET'S START

1. Put salad leaves, coriander leaves, ginger, garlic, peppercorns, lemon juice and salt in a blender and churn well.
2. Keep the tomato wedges and the julienned spring onions in a bowl.
3. Pour the blended green sauce over the mixture.
4. Toss well so that each wedge is brushed with the sauce.
5. Serve with any meal and skip cereals.

IMMUNE POWER

Surprisingly pleasant! Tender turnips taste as sweet as carrot and are a super food for the mucous membranes, really building your child's immunity with every bite.

INGREDIENTS

1. 2 carrots, medium
2. 1 radish, medium
3. 1 turnip, medium
4. 2 Indian gooseberry or 2 tsp lemon juice
5. 1 tsp yellow mustard seeds
6. ½ tsp bishop's weed
7. 2 black peppercorns
8. Black salt to taste

GETTING READY

1. Wash, scrape and cut into juliennes carrot, radish and turnip.
2. Grate the gooseberries and put all in a jar.
3. Grind the mustard seeds, bishop's weed and pepper corns coarsely.

LET'S START

1. Sprinkle the ground spices on the vegetables in the jar.
2. Add salt to taste.
3. If you are using lemon juice, then add it now. Cover the jar and shake well.
4. Keep in sun for 8-10 hours to extract full flavours from the vegetables.
5. Refrigerate and use in next meal.
6. Enjoy the piquant salad.

ENERGY REVIVER

INGREDIENTS

1. 2 carrots, medium
2. 1 beetroot, medium
3. 1 spring onion
4. 1 cucumber, medium
5. 40 peanuts, raw
6. Sea salt to taste
7. Lemon juice to taste

NOTE
Whenever spring onions are not available, you can substitute with the common red onions that are on sale throughout the year.

Gustatory! Appeals to all the senses and builds blood. Strengthens the body and raises the haemoglobin. A boon for anaemic children.

GETTING READY

1. Soak raw peanuts overnight. Remove the pink skin and chop coarsely.
2. Wash and scrape carrot and beetroot. Shred the carrot and chop beetroot into very small pieces.
3. Peel cucumber and dice along with spring onion.

LET'S START

1. Put all vegetables in a salad bowl.
2. Sprinkle chopped peanuts from top and add sea salt. Mix lightly.
3. Squeeze lemon juice to dress the salad.
4. Refrigerate for a while if desired.

DREAM SALAD

INGREDIENTS

1. 2 red cabbage leaves
2. 6 pieces baby corn, fresh
3. 1 spring onion
4. 2 pieces coconut chunks (2" each), fresh
5. 4-6 karoundas
6. ¼ tsp bishop's weed
7. ¼ tsp fennel seeds
8. Black salt to taste

A glorious salad with strong flavours. Potent with concentrated phytochemicals, this salad will go well with a light meal. Allow the body to get full benefits by consuming it with the food.

GETTING READY

1. Wash all vegetables well before using.
2. Soak cabbage leaves in salt water for 30 minutes. Rinse and shred through a grater.
3. Chop spring onion, its green stalk and the baby corns finely.
4. Scrape the brown skin of the coconut chunks and chop.

LET'S START

1. Keep shredded cabbage, chopped onion and baby corns in a bowl.
2. In a blender take the karoundas and add coconut, bishop's weed, fennel seeds and salt.
3. Churn to make a smooth and creamy sauce.
4. Spoon this sauce over the vegetables in the bowl.
5. Toss lightly to mix in the flavours.
6. Relish this dreamy salad before starting your meal.

SECRET OF ANGELS

INGREDIENTS

1. 4 red radish
2. 1 red lettuce, full head
3. 2 carrots
4. 1 yellow bell pepper
5. Few mint leaves, fresh
6. 1 tsp cumin seeds
7. 2 tsp sesame seeds
8. 2 tsp lemon juice
9. Black salt to taste

This is a salad we experimented with to get a good amount of minerals, vitamins, chlorophyll and fibre in children's diet. The good part is that children don't get bored of it since the colours can keep changing. Use red or green lettuce, red or orange carrots, red or white radish, and you will have a different salad everytime.

GETTING READY

1. Wash and soak sesame seeds in water for 6-8 hours. Drain water.
2. Lightly roast cumin seeds and grind them.
3. Wash all vegetables and cut radish, carrots and yellow bell pepper in juliennes.
4. Chop red lettuce leaves and mint leaves.

LET'S START

1. Put radish, carrots, bell pepper and red lettuce in a bowl.
2. Grind mint leaves with sesame seeds along with salt and lemon juice.
3. Add mint cream to the vegetables in a bowl. Toss lightly.
4. Sprinkle cumin powder on top.
5. Serve before main meal.

KNOCK OUT

The goodness of coconut is in its creaminess when blended making the perfect dressing. Tastes better than mayonnaise and gives 100 per cent nutrition. You just can't beat it.

INGREDIENTS

1. 1 red bell pepper, medium
2. 1 onion
3. 2 carrots
4. A small chunk of coconut, fresh
5. 1 pod garlic
6. 1/4" ginger root, fresh
7. ½" stick cinnamon
8. 2 black pepper corns
9. Lemon juice to taste
10. ½ tsp extra virgin olive oil
11. Black salt to taste

GETTING READY

1. Wash and chop bell pepper, carrots and onion in desired size and shape.
2. Scrape the brown skin of the coconut chunk.

LET'S START

1. Keep chopped vegetables in a salad bowl.
2. In a blender put coconut chunk, ginger, garlic, extra virgin olive oil and the spices.
3. Grind to paste. Season with salt, add lemon juice if required.
4. Dress up vegetables in the bowl with the coconut sauce.
5. Chill for 10 minutes before serving.

LONDON SPECIAL

INGREDIENTS

1. 1 iceberg lettuce, full head
2. ½ beetroot
3. 1 cup sweet corn
4. 1 green chilli
5. ½ tsp extra virgin olive oil
6. Lemon juice to taste

Iceberg lettuce is the king of lettuces with its clean, crispy texture. Known to cleanse the blood and an excellent food for the joints, it is the key ingredient in this salad while sweet corn plays the delicious counterpart.

GETTING READY

1. Wash iceberg lettuce under running water. Any speck of dust on the leaves put you off.
2. Tear the lettuce into bite size pieces.
3. Wash, scrape and chop beetroot.

LET'S START

1. In a pan, steam the sweet corn for 3-4 minutes.
2. Put the sweet corn and the iceberg pieces into a bowl.
3. Blend beetroot, olive oil, and green chilli along with lemon juice into a paste.
4. Mix the blended dressing into the corn and lettuce.
5. Serve this hearty salad before the main meal.

PERFECT 10

This salad scores the perfect ten on nutrition and wholesomeness. It can be eaten as a meal itself or with another dry vegetable to round it off.

INGREDIENTS

1. 500 gm boneless chicken
2. 500 gm shelled peas
3. 2 garlic pods
4. ½" ginger root, fresh
5. Few sprigs of coriander leaves, fresh
6. 10 black pepper corns
7. 1 tsp lemon juice or tamarind juice
8. 1 tsp extra virgin olive oil
9. Salt to taste

GETTING READY

1. Grind the black pepper corns coarsely.
2. Sliver the chicken in long pieces.
3. Wash the shelled peas and coriander leaves.
4. Crush the ginger and garlic to take out juice.

LET'S START

1. In a non-stick pan, sauté the chicken slivers and the green peas till tender.
2. Season with salt and ground black pepper.
3. Add juice of ginger and garlic.
4. Switch off flame and pour lemon juice or tamarind juice on top.
5. Transfer to serving dish and garnish with chopped coriander leaves.

PARISIAN SALAD

INGREDIENTS

1. 4 leaves, green cabbage
2. 3 tsp sprouted brown chick peas
3. 1 onion, medium
4. 1 green chilli
5. ½" ginger root, fresh
6. Few coriander leaves, fresh
7. 1 ½ tsp hung curd
8. 1 tsp black mustard seeds
9. Black salt to taste

Black gram has been known for centuries for stamina building and combining it with a touch of yoghurt brings out an exotic flavour altogether. Totally tantalizes the taste buds!

GETTING READY

1. Wash and soak cabbage leaves in salt water for 30 minutes. Rinse and chop leaves very finely.
2. Crush black gram sprouts with a rolling pin.
3. Wash and chop onion and coriander leaves.
4. Grind ginger and chilli and mix in hung curd.
5. Grind mustard seeds and keep aside.

LET'S START

1. Keep the cabbage leaves in a bowl.
2. Add coarsely crushed sprouts, chopped onion and coriander leaves.
3. Spoon the hung curd in the bowl and toss to mix well.
4. Add salt and ground mustard seeds and mix again.
5. Parisian style salad is ready to serve.

WHIZZ BANG

INGREDIENTS

1. 2 carrots
2. 1 red bell pepper, small
3. 5 spinach leaves, tender
4. 15 cherry tomatoes
5. 1 green chilli
6. 3 garlic pods
7. 2 tsp sunflower seeds
8. 1 tsp lemon juice
9. Salt to taste

Cherry tomatoes have that unique taste not found in ordinary tomatoes and with sunflower seeds they make this absolutely delectable creamy sauce. Spinach adds the extra iron making this salad an unbeatable accompaniment to your child's meal.

GETTING READY

1. Wash, scrape gently and cut carrots into juliennes.
2. De-core the bell pepper, wash and mince finely. Put both in a bowl.
3. Wash the spinach leaves in warm salty water and chop finely.
4. Wash seeds, tomatoes and peel the garlic pods.

LET'S START

1. In a blender, put the cherry tomatoes, green chilli, garlic pods, lemon juice and the sunflower seeds. Churn to make a smooth paste.
2. Add finely chopped spinach leaves to the sauce.
3. Pour this creamy sauce over the julienned carrots and the minced red bell pepper.
4. Toss lightly to mix in well.
5. Serve fresh with the main meal.

5 EVENING RECHARGERS

BLOOD DETOX

INGREDIENTS

1. 1 pomegranate, deep red variety
2. 1 apple
3. A handful of mint leaves, fresh
4. ½ ginger root, fresh
5. A pinch of cinnamon powder

A literal blood builder and cleanser, this juice is unbeatable in taste. Its health building properties make this a terrific option to give after your children come back from playing.

GETTING READY

1. Choose and pick a deep red skin pomegranate. Wash and cut into four parts and take out the ruby coloured kernels.
2. Wash and scrub apple. Core out the seeds and slice apple without peeling.
3. Peel and wash ginger.
4. Wash mint leaves under running tap water.

LET'S START

1. Put all ingredients except the cinnamon through the juicer.
2. Pour extracted juice in a glass.
3. Stir in cinnamon powder.
4. Serve immediately.

TASTE BUBBLE

INGREDIENTS

1. 500 gm raw papaya
2. ½ ginger root, fresh
3. 1 lemon
4. Palm candy to taste

If you have never tasted raw papaya juice, then you have missed one of the tastiest juices the vegetable world has to offer. Similar in taste to carrot juice with its unique flavour, this is food fit for Gods.

GETTING READY

1. Pick a deep green, fresh papaya taking care not to pick one with shrivelled skin.
2. Wash and peel raw papaya taking care to remove the entire dark green skin. Cut into half and remove the white covering by scraping it off.
3. Wash the papaya in liberal water and cut into thin slices.
4. Peel ginger and wash.

LET'S START

1. Put raw papaya slices through the juicer.
2. Put ginger through the juicer, too.
3. Pour in a glass and squeeze juice of a lemon.
4. Add palm candy.
5. Stir well to dissolve palm candy.
6. Serve chilled by adding some crushed ice if your child likes cold drinks.
7. Drink without waiting since nutrients can get oxidized.

SWEET 'N' MAGICAL

A divine invitation to the tongue! These come out like chocolate and the kids can never have enough of them. Keep them locked or you won't know when they get kidnapped.

INGREDIENTS

1. 200 gm soya flour
2. 200 gm white oats
3. 100 gm gram flour
4. ½ coconut, fresh
5. 5 apricots, dried
6. 20 pieces munakka
7. ½ tsp cinnamon powder

GETTING READY

1. Soak dry apricots and munakka in just level water for 2 hours.
2. Break open coconut, keep water aside.
3. Scrape brown skin and desiccate coconut.

LET'S START

1. Roast gram flour and soya flour on slow flame for 8-10 minutes.
2. Blend coconut, munakka and apricots in a food blender to a creamy consistency.
3. Add coconut water, if required.
4. Turn this cream into a broad shallow container.
5. Add to it gram flour mixture along with white oats. Mix with hand to evenly distribute all ingredients.
6. Add cinnamon powder. Mix again properly.
7. Press hard and make the surface smooth level. Cut into 3-4" long and 1" wide pieces.
8. Wrap them in silver foil or wax paper.
9. Refrigerate them.
10. Children will love these natural energizing 'chocolates'.

> **NOTE**
> Gram flour is flour made from ground brown chick peas. Commonly known as 'besan' in Hindi, it is widely used in Indian cooking.

SWEET BLESSINGS

INGREDIENTS

1. 200 gm gram flour
2. 40 pieces dates, black variety
3. 2 tsp poppy seeds
4. 10 almonds
5. 1 tsp melon seeds
6. 2" chunk of coconut, fresh

A power house of nutrition, made with nuts, seeds, dates and gram flour – all nutrient dense foods, this snack can resurrect the dead so to say. A veritable blessing for growing kids.

GETTING READY

1. Soak almonds for 5-6 hrs. Peel almonds and chop them coarsely.
2. Wash and de-seed dates. Chop dates finely.
3. Dice coconut into small pieces.
4. Wash melon seeds, drain water and crush them.

LET'S START

1. Roast gram flour on slow flame till it is golden brown.
2. Grind dates and coconut together adding part of roasted gram flour to blend dates well.
3. Combine minced dates and balance roasted gram flour, almonds and melon seeds. Make a homogenous mixture by using pressure of hand.
4. Make small balls and mould them into 2" cylindrical shape.
5. Roll them in semi-roasted poppy seeds to give them outer texture, taste and nutrition.
6. Refrigerate them to get a crunchy taste.

CHILDREN'S FAVOURITE

INGREDIENTS

1. 6-8 stalks of lemon grass (4" length), fresh
2. 1 tsp lemon juice
3. ½ tsp honey
4. 250 ml water

> **NOTE**
> You can also use dried lemon grass herb of equal quantity when fresh is not available.

The tangy flavour and the potency of lemon grass will make it your child's favourite. Great for improving digestion, children love it cold. Chill and serve as an iced tea in summers.

GETTING READY

1. Wash the freshly cut lemon grass and chop the stalks.

LET'S START

1. Put them in a pan. Pour the water in the pan and let it boil.
2. Turn off the flame. Allow the leaves to steep in it for minimum 10 minutes.
3. Squeeze in juice of one whole lemon and stir in rock candy.
4. Strain and pour the blend in your cup to sip it warm.

IMMUNITY RAISER

Holy basil leaves are a nerve tonic and help sharpen memory. Your child's nervous system will remain healthy with clear and vibrant signals. The leaves raise immunity and resistance to pollutants. Its regular intake has a marvelous effect on children.

INGREDIENTS

1. 15 -20 holy basil leaves, fresh
2. 4 pepper corns
3. 1/4th tsp dry ginger
4. ½ tsp honey
5. 200 ml water

GETTING READY

1. Wash the holy basil leaves thoroughly under running tap water and chop them finely.
2. Coarsely crush pepper corns.
3. Grind dry ginger into a powder.

LET'S START

1. Put water in a pan and add finely chopped holy basil leaves to the pan.
2. Put it on flame to boil.
3. Add pepper corns and dry ginger powder.
4. Boil it for 2 to 3 minutes.
5. Strain into your cup and stir in the honey.

NOTE
A wonder drink to give during colds, coughs and viral fevers. It will give relief almost instantly.

INFUSE YOUR IMMUNITY

INGREDIENTS

1. 1 ½" stick cinnamon
2. ½ tsp black cumin seeds
3. ½ tsp honey
4. 200 ml water

Black cumin has been used by millions of people for its immunity enhancing properties.

It stimulates the bone marrow and immune cells to function better. Cinnamon boosts cognitive function and memory capacity.

GETTING READY

Wash the cinnamon stick and break it into small pieces.

LET'S START

1. Take water in a pan and boil it.
2. Put the pounded cinnamon in the boiling water along with black cumin seeds.
3. Cover the pan and allow it to boil for 2 minutes. Put off the flame.
4. Keep it covered for a while to allow the infusion of cinnamon and black cumin seeds to blend well.
5. Put clear honey in your cup and strain the infusion into it. Stir to mix in the honey.
6. Serve a cup or two in the evenings without any other snack.

6 MAGIC MEALS

All the following meals have been designed using foods effective in strengthening the immune system. These meals can be served on weekends to children. We have given 9 magic meals so that in a month, eight of the combinations given will be served without repeating even a single one. This will ensure a balanced nutritional intake as well as a change of flavours, tastes, aromas and texture in food. You can choose each meal according to your child's preference; they are not given in any order. Keep in mind that these meals give good results only when they are served as is without making any addition or substitution.

A salad from the Salad Pot section will be served with these feasts. You will be choosing the salad as given in the '12 weeks immunity plan' to serve on weekends.

Feast one: A new 'kid tested' way of making French beans served with gravy styled green peas. The accompanying wholesome and hearty multi grain rotis make this a feast for the taste buds.

CRUNCH MUNCHY BEANS

INGREDIENTS

1. 250 gm french beans
2. 1 tomato, red and ripe
3. 1 onion
4. 4 cloves
5. ½ tsp dry ginger powder

GETTING READY

1. Grind all spices together and keep aside.
2. Wash, de-thread and cut beans into 1" pieces.
3. Wash and chop tomatoes finely.
4. Peel and chop onion.

6. 1 tsp coriander seeds
7. 10 black pepper corns
8. 1 brown cardamom, large
9. ¾ tsp fennel seeds
10. 1" cinnamon stick
11. ¾ tsp salt
12. 1 tsp lemon juice
13. 1 tsp extra virgin olive oil
14. Water as required

LET'S START

1. Boil water, put salt and drop beans in it. Cover the pan.
2. Put off the flame. Keep beans covered for 10 minutes.
3. Strain water.
4. Put oil in a pan and immediately add chopped onions. Within a minute stir in french beans, chopped tomatoes and ground spices.
5. Add salt to taste.
6. Cover pan and cook till beans are crunchy and tender.
7. Pour lemon juice just before serving.

HOT SHOT PEAS

INGREDIENTS

1. 100 gm baby corn, tender with soft core
2. 1 green bell pepper, large
3. 350 gm green peas, fresh and unshelled
4. 1 carrot, large
5. 1 onion, large
6. 50 gm coriander leaves, fresh
7. 4 garlic pods
8. 1 green chilli
9. 1 tsp coriander powder
10. 1 tsp extra virgin olive oil
11. Juice of one lemon
12. Salt to taste

NOTE
Baby corn is also known as candle corn in Thai cuisine. It's from the maize family and is the soft ears, handpicked in the farm. These are eaten whole that means cob included, whereas in mature corn only kernels are eaten. Baby corns can be eaten raw in salads or mildly cooked only.

GETTING READY

1. Shell peas.
2. Wash baby corn in lukewarm salted water. Cut baby corn in diagonals, each ¼th of an inch.
3. Wash and chop green bell pepper in ½ inch squares.
4. Wash and chop carrot, coriander leaves and green chilli.
5. Peel and chop onion and garlic coarsely.
6. In a blender, add onion, carrot, garlic, chilli and coriander leaves and grind together.

LET'S START

1. Put oil in a pan and pour the above ground mixture in it. Cover the pan and simmer on slow flame.
2. Stir and add salt and coriander powder. Cover pan again and simmer for 5 minutes.
3. Add shelled peas and baby corn diagonals. Cover the pan and cook till both are tender.
4. Add chopped bell pepper. Stir and simmer for another few minutes taking care to retain the colour of the bell pepper.
5. Switch off flame and transfer to a serving bowl.
6. Squeeze lemon juice from top.
7. Serve piping hot.

MULTI GRAIN ROTIS

INGREDIENTS

1. 1 cup barley flour
2. ½ cup whole wheat flour
3. 1 tsp extra virgin olive oil
4. water as required

GETTING READY

1. Mix both flours together in a kneading utensil.
2. Knead the flour gradually adding water to make smooth and soft dough.

LET'S START

1. Make equal parts of dough. Roll out rotis by placing a ball of dough on a clean transparent poly-sheet.
2. First press it with hands to flatten as much as you can. Finally put another sheet on it and use a rolling pin to make it larger and thinner rotis.
3. Cook on a non-stick girddle on a medium flame.
4. Apply extra virgin olive oil.
5. You will get approximately four rotis.

FLAVOURED BABY POTATOES

INGREDIENTS

1. 300 gm baby potatoes, small ½"- ¾" size
2. 2" coconut chunk, fresh
3. 1 carrot, small
4. Few mint leaves, fresh
5. 1 tsp oregano, dried
6. ½ tsp mustard seeds
7. 50 gm tamarind, dried
8. Black salt to taste
9. 1 tsp extra virgin olive oil
10. 75 ml purified water

Feast two: *The goodness of whole wheat rotis served with tempting baby potatoes flavoured with mint. But it is the pumpkin in this meal which makes its mark as the food for immunity.*

GETTING READY

1. Soak tamarind in warm water for 1-2 hours. Mash tamarind to extract pulp. Strain and keep aside.
2. Coarsely grind mustard seeds.
3. Wash potatoes well and semi-boil them in salt water along with the skin.
4. Peel or scrape brown skin of coconut.
5. Scoop out the eyes of carrot and scrape.
6. Grate carrot and coconut.
7. Wash and chop mint leaves and keep aside.

LET'S START

1. Peel the skin of potatoes. Rub a mixture of salt and oregano on them.
2. Grease the tray with oil and place potatoes.
3. Grill potatoes for 10-15 minutes in a preheated oven.
4. To check they are cooked poke a toothpick in the center of a potato. If it passes smoothly, potatoes are done.
5. Combine tamarind pulp, grated carrot, coconut, salt and ground mustard seeds. Mix them well using a rolling and tossing movement.
6. Lace this salad on the base of a boat shape shallow bowl.
7. Top the salad with grilled potatoes.
8. Dress with chopped mint leaves and serve.

THE PUMPKIN WIZARD

INGREDIENTS

1. 500 gm green pumpkin
2. 1 red bell pepper, large
3. 10 green olives (optional)
4. 2 green chillies
5. 4 garlic pods
6. 4 spinach leaves, tender
7. 1 tsp black mustard seeds, ground
8. ½ tsp fenugreek seeds
9. A pinch of nutmeg powder
10. A pinch of asafoetida
11. 1 tsp extra virgin olive oil
12. Salt to taste

NOTE
Pumpkin is available in green, yellow and red variety. This recipe uses only the green variety which is usually consumed with its nutrient rich skin. If desired, you can mash some of the pumpkin cubes to get a more fluid texture.

GETTING READY

24 hours before:
1. Wash and de-core red bell pepper and dice.
2. Slit green chillies.
3. Cut olives.
4. Rub a mixture of salt and mustard powder on the above ingredients. Place them in a tight jar and keep them in the sun for a day.

At the time of preparation:
1. Wash and cut pumpkin. Remove the seeds and chop into 1" cubes retaining the skin.
2. Wash spinach leaves in salt water and shred them.
3. Peel and chop garlic finely.

LET'S START

1. Put pan on a low flame. Add oil, fenugreek seeds and asafoetida. As fenugreek starts changing colour, add chopped garlic.
2. Stir and add cubes of pumpkin and salt. Stir again and cover the pan. Cook till tender.
3. Add spiced bell pepper, olives and green chillies.
4. Flavour it with a pinch of nutmeg.
5. Put off the flame but keep the pan covered to allow the flavours and tastes to mix in and get soaked in the vegetable.
6. Transfer the dish to a bowl and dress the pumpkin with finely chopped spinach leaves.
7. Serve hot.

WHOLE WHEAT ROTIS

INGREDIENTS

1. 1 ½ cup whole wheat flour
2. Extra virgin olive oil
3. Water as required

GETTING READY

1. Take the flour in a kneading utensil.
2. Knead the flour gradually adding water to make a smooth and soft dough.

LET'S START

1. Roll out into thin rotis using a rolling pin to make large rotis. Use butter paper as a base to avoid them from sticking on the surface, if required.
2. Cook them on a non-stick griddle.
3. Apply extra virgin olive oil.
4. 4 Delicious rotis will be ready to be feasted on.

SEA FEST

INGREDIENTS

1. 150 gm shelled prawns
2. 1 onion, large
3. 1 cucumber, small
4. 1" ginger root, fresh
5. 6 garlic pods
6. Few sprigs of parsley, fresh
7. Few mint leaves, fresh
8. 2 bay leaves
9. ½ tsp garam masala
10. 4 black pepper corns
11. 1 tsp extra virgin olive oil
12. Few lemon wedges
13. Salt to taste

Feast three: *The culmination of research, prawns is the gift from the sea for supporting the immune system and what a delightful way to do it. The zucchini balances the meal in nutrients and the power grain rotis add a whole new dimension to the feast.*

GETTING READY

1. Shell and clean the prawns. Devein them with care.
2. Wash, peel and cut the onion in long slices.
3. Peel and cube cucumber, put it in a bowl.
4. Make paste of ginger, garlic, parsley, mint leaves and pepper corns.
5. Squeeze in lemon juice.
6. Toss cucumber in this sauce.

LET'S START

1. Heat oil in a sauce pan.
2. Add bay leaves, onion and prawns, and stir very gently for 4-5 minutes.
3. Sprinkle salt and garam masala and stir. Cover to cook till prawns are tender.
4. Switch off the flame and add the above prepared spice sauce with tossed cucumber into the saucepan.
5. Gently mix in spicy sauce into cooked prawns.
6. Arrange more lemon wedges on top before serving.

> **NOTE**
>
> Use fresh prawns whenever possible. Frozen prawns are also easy to use and available commercially in all good stores and malls.
>
> Adjust the level of spices and the quantity of garam masala according to your child's taste.

BOWL OF LIFE

INGREDIENTS

1. 1 yellow zucchini or green zucchini
2. 100 gm red beans, fresh
3. 50 gm baby corn, tender with soft cores
4. 1 yellow bell pepper
5. 1 spring onion
6. 1 green chilli
7. 1 tsp juice of garlic
8. 1 tsp extra virgin olive oil
9. Salt to taste

GETTING READY

1. Scrape zucchini very gently. Cut zucchini in julienne shape.
2. Wash and de-thread red beans. Cut red beans 1" long.
3. Wash baby corn in salt water. Cut baby corn in 4 long sections and make them 1" long.
4. Wash and deseed yellow bell pepper, cut into julienne.
5. Cut spring onion and its green stalk into julienne.
6. Cut green chillies into four long pieces.

LET'S START

1. Put oil in a pan.
2. Stir in beans, zucchini and salt. Cover pan and cook till beans are tender and zucchini is almost soft.
3. Add onion, bell pepper, baby corn, green chillies and juice of garlic.
4. Stir the vegetables and cover the pan tightly.
5. Cook on slow flame for 3-4 minutes.
6. Put off the flame. Keep the pan covered for a while.
7. Serve hot.

NOTE

There can be times when fresh red beans are not available. Substitute with sword beans or cluster beans. The benefits of this recipe are lost without beans as an ingredient. In Indian translation, zucchini's are tori but actually they are a different squash vegetable available in green and yellow colour.

POWER GRAIN ROTIS

INGREDIENTS

1. 1 cup whole wheat flour
2. ½ cup gram flour
3. 1 tsp extra virgin olive oil
4. Water as required

GETTING READY

1. Mix both flours together in a kneading utensil.
2. Knead the flour gradually adding water to make smooth and soft dough.

LET'S START

1. Make equal parts of the dough.
2. Roll out rotis by placing the ball of dough on a clean transparent poly-sheet.
3. First press the ball with hands to flatten as much as you can. Finally put another sheet on it and use a rolling pin to make it a larger and thinner roti.
4. Cook on non-stick girdle on a medium flame.
5. Apply extra virgin olive oil.
6. You will get approximately four rotis.

VINTAGE BIRYANI

INGREDIENTS

1. 1 cup unpolished rice or brown rice
2. 50 gm peas, shelled
3. 2 florets of cauliflower
4. 1 carrot, small
5. 5 french beans
6. 1 onion
7. 2 green chillies
8. 1" ginger root, fresh
9. 1" turmeric root, fresh
10. 1 tsp caraway seeds
11. 2 green cardamoms
12. 1 bay leaf
13. 1 tsp extra virgin olive oil
14. Salt to taste
15. 50 ml water

NOTE

Brown rice needs to be soaked for at least two hours before cooking as the grains of brown rice are tougher than the white rice. This helps in its easy cooking.

Feast four: If there has ever been a favourite with kids, it is the biryani. Served here with a mouthwatering yoghurt raita, your children will be left licking their fingers.

GETTING READY

1. Wash and soak rice for 8-10 hours.
2. Wash and soak cauliflower in salt water for 30 minutes. Drain and cut cauliflower into small florets.
3. Wash, gently scrape and cut carrot into small cubes.
4. Wash, peel and chop onion and ginger into juliennes.
5. Chop green chillies and turmeric very finely and then crush with a roller pin.
6. Wash, de-thread beans and chop as fine as green chilies.
7. Grind caraway seeds, cardamoms and bay leaf into fine powder.
8. Wash shelled peas once before using.

LET'S START

1. Put oil in a non-stick pressure cooker and at the same time, add onion and ginger. Cook for a while on a slow flame.
2. Add peas and cauliflower florets. Cover cooker without whistle and cook for 2 minutes.
3. Stir and add the remaining vegetables. Stir and cook for a minute.
4. Add rice, salt, ground spices and water. Stir and cover cooker.
5. Give one whistle and put off the flame.
6. Let the pressure reduce on its own allowing the vegetables to get steamed and the spices to blend in.
7. Serve hot with yoghurt raita.

Magic Meals 177

GATE TO HEALTH

INGREDIENTS

1. 500 gm yoghurt
2. 100 gm florets of broccoli
3. 1 yellow bell pepper
4. 1 spring onion
5. ½" ginger root, fresh
6. A handful mint leaves, fresh
7. Few coriander sprigs, fresh
8. 1 green chilli
9. ½ tsp roasted cumin, grounded
10. Black salt to taste

GETTING READY

1. Wash mint leaves and chop them very finely.
2. Set yogurt overnight along with chopped mint.
3. Cut head of broccoli and make small florets and put them in salt water for 30 minutes. Strain them.
4. Separately heat water in a pan to boiling point. Put off the flame.
5. Dip broccoli florets in hot water and immediately pass them through ice cold water and strain.
6. Wash yellow bell pepper taking care to rub crevices.
7. Open, remove seeds and dice the bell pepper.
8. Peel and chop onion finely along with the green stalk.
9. Wash and chop coriander leaves, ginger and green chilli.
10. Keep the diced bell pepper and chopped onion in a bowl separately.

LET'S START

1. Put ginger, coriander sprigs, broccoli and green chilli in the blender and churn twice.
2. Add mint flavoured yoghurt to the blender and churn it once only.
3. Add black salt and cumin powder.
4. Pour the smooth and creamy green mixture into the bowl consisting of yellow bell pepper and onion.
5. Serve cool or chilled in summers.

TURNIP SOUP

INGREDIENTS

1. 1 carrot, medium
2. 1 turnip, large
3. 2 red cabbage leaves
4. 1 spring onion
5. 2 cloves
6. ¼ tsp white pepper or to taste
7. 3 cups water
8. Rock Salt to taste

Feast five: *A soup for the soul, literally, served with exotic lotus roots made with spices. Wheat used with the endosperm is used for the rotis accompanying this meal.*

GETTING READY

1. Wash and gently scrape the carrot and turnip.
2. Rinse cabbage leaves in plain water and soak them in salt water for 30 minutes. Drain them.
3. Peel the spring onion.
4. Chop carrot, turnip, cabbage and spring onion.
5. Chop green stalks of spring onion and keep them separately.

LET'S START

1. Cook chopped vegetables in water on slow flame. Keep pan covered and simmer till vegetables are tender.
2. Add salt and sieve soup.
3. Transfer to a blender and add cloves. Blend vegetables to a smooth consistency.
4. Strain if you choose to. Sprinkle pepper and stir.
5. Pour in a soup bowl.
6. Garnish the hot soup with the chopped green stalk of spring onions just before serving.

HEALING ROOTS

INGREDIENTS

For roots:

1. 2 lotus roots, full length
2. 1 tsp turmeric powder
3. 2 tsp aniseed powder
4. 1 tsp cumin seed powder
5. ½ tsp black pepper powder
6. ½ tsp black cardamom powder
7. 3 green cardamom, powdered
8. Salt to taste

For main:

1. 1 head broccoli, medium
2. 4 tomatoes, red and ripe
3. 1 spring onion or red onion
4. 1 green chilli
5. 4-5 cloves
6. A pinch of asafoetida
7. 2 tsp extra virgin olive oil

GETTING READY

For roots:

1. Scrape the roots gently taking care to remove the darkened skin. Cut off the end points.
2. Run pressurized water through the holes of the lotus root to remove every speck of mud.
3. Drain and dry completely the lotus root from outside.
4. Cut into ½" diagonal pieces and spread them on a clean plate.
5. Make a mixture of all the dry spices and fill in the root holes.

For main:

1. Wash and break broccoli into florets. Scrape and chop the stem. Soak in warm salted water for half an hour. Drain water.
2. Peel and chop onion and garlic.
3. Wash and chop tomatoes.
4. In a blender, add broccoli stem pieces, onion, garlic, green chilli and tomatoes. Grind to a paste.

LET'S START

For roots:

1. Put oil in a pressure cooker and add 2 tsp of water.
2. Carefully pick each piece of spiced lotus root and place in the pressure cooker.
3. Close the lid and cook for two whistles.

NOTE

Lotus root must be picked up with care. Each root should have a sealed top and end; else there will be too much mud too clean and this can be cumbersome.

The lotus root is a crunchy vegetable found to be rich in dietary fibre, vitamin C, potassium, thiamine, ribo-flavin, vitamin B6, phosphorus, copper, and manganese. You must make it a regular part of your children's nutritional intake.

For main:

1. In a pan, boil 300 ml of water. Add broccoli florets and ½ tsp salt.
2. Cover the pan and put off the flame. Allow it to remain for a minute. Drain the water completely.
3. Open the pressure cooker and add the ground mixture of broccoli stem and tomatoes. Close the lid and give one more whistle or till lotus root becomes tender.
4. Next, add the broccoli florets to the lotus root. Toss well and cover the lid for 5 minutes.
5. Transfer to a serving dish.

WHOLE WHEAT ROTIS

INGREDIENTS

1. 1 ½ cup whole wheat flour
2. Extra virgin olive oil
3. Water as required

GETTING READY

1. Take the flour in a kneading utensil.
2. Knead the flour by gradually adding water to make smooth and soft dough.

LET'S START

1. Roll out into thin rotis using a rolling pin to make large and thin rotis.
2. Use butter paper as base to avoid them sticking on the surface if required.
3. Cook them on a non-stick griddle.
4. Apply extra virgin olive oil.
5. 4 delicious rotis will be ready to be feasted on.

CELERY SOUP

INGREDIENTS

1. 2 stalks of celery
2. 100 gm peas, fresh and unshelled
3. 1 tsp thyme herb, dried
4. 2 spring onions
5. ¾ ginger root, fresh
6. 2 garlic pods or green garlic, when available
7. 1 lemon
8. ½ tsp ground mustard seeds
9. Salt to taste
10. 3 cups purified water

NOTE
Celery is a unique combination of tastes – salty with a dash of bitter. It is loaded with antioxidants and is highly nutritious. The stalks are used in cooking while the leaves are to be removed.

Feast six: There are few soups which can compare in taste with this celery soup. Served here with a medley of sweet corn and cabbage along with a special roti made with onions.

GETTING READY

1. Remove leaves of celery and chop stalks only.
2. Smear salt and ground mustard seeds. Cover and keep aside for 20 minutes.
3. Shell peas. Wash peas once.
4. Wash, peel and chop onion with its greens, ginger and garlic.
5. Wash chopped celery stalks with plain water.

LET'S START

1. In a pan, heat water to less than boiling point and put off the flame.
2. Add all the chopped vegetables, green peas, salt and thyme.
3. Cook on a low flame for 3-4 minutes. Put off the flame. Cover the pan. Leave for 8-10 minutes.
4. Transfer all contents of pan to a blender and churn well.
5. Sieve the blended soup.
6. Squeeze lemon juice before serving for that tangy taste.
7. Serve warm.

ENRAPTURE

INGREDIENTS

1. 1 green cabbage, small head
2. 1 corn on the cob, full ear
3. 3 spring onions
4. 2 tomatoes, medium, ripe and red
5. 2 garlic pods
6. 1 green chilli
7. Few leaves of coriander leaves, fresh
8. ½ tsp cumin seeds
9. 1 green cardamom
10. 1 tsp coriander powder
11. A pinch of cinnamon powder
12. 2 tsp extra virgin olive oil
13. Salt to taste

NOTE
Vegetables turn out more tasty when the ingredients used are fresh and of deep colour. Make it a practice to use fully ripe, deep red tomatoes to get their full flavour. You are encouraged to make these dishes throughout the year, so if any ingredient is not available like spring onions, go ahead and substitute with common red onions that you do have.

GETTING READY

1. Wash cabbage leaves and soak in salt water for 30 minutes. Shred the cabbage.
2. Remove kernels from the corn cob.
3. Peel and slice onions into thin slivers.
4. Wash rest of the vegetables including the remaining green stalks of the onions.
5. In a blender, grind green stalks, garlic, chilli, tomatoes and green cardamom.

LET'S START

1. Put oil in a pan. Add cumin seeds and allow them to change colour.
2. Add sliced onions and cook till they turn translucent.
3. Add the ground tomato mixture, stir and cover pan. Cook on a low flame for 5-6 minutes.
4. Add shredded cabbage, salt and cinnamon.
5. Cover the pan and cook on a low flame till cabbage becomes tender and yet retains its colour.
6. Transfer to a bowl.
7. Garnish with coriander leaves before serving.

ROTI DO PYAZA

INGREDIENTS

1. 2 onions
2. 1 ½ cup whole wheat flour
3. Extra virgin Olive oil
4. Water as required

NOTE
You can use spring onions when they are in season. Remember to use the green stalks as well since the stalk contains many nutrients including chlorophyll.

GETTING READY

1. Wash, peel and chop onions very finely.
2. Take the flour and onions in a kneading utensil.
3. Knead the flour by gradually adding water to make smooth and soft dough.

LET'S START

1. Roll out into thin rotis using a rolling pin to make large and thin rotis.
2. Use butter paper as base to avoid them sticking on the surface if required.
3. Cook them on a non-stick griddle.
4. Apply extra virgin olive oil.
5. 4 delicious rotis will be ready to serve your loved ones.

FIT FOR CHAMPIONS

INGREDIENTS

1. 1 cup green mung beans, dried
2. 4 tomatoes, large, red and ripe
3. 2 onions
4. 1" ginger root, fresh
5. 8 garlic pods
6. Few sprigs of coriander leaves, fresh
7. 1-2 green chillies to taste
8. 1 tsp cumin seeds
9. 1 tsp coriander powder
10. ½ tsp red chilli powder (optional)
11. 3 tsp extra virgin olive oil
12. Salt to taste

Feast seven: Mung beans made in the 'dal makhani' style and a new look bottle gourd recipe are the heart of this feast. The rotis are a surprise with a stuffing of cabbage.

GETTING READY

1. Wash and soak mung beans for 4-5 hours.
2. Wash, peel and chop onions.
3. Wash and puree tomatoes separately.
4. Mince ginger, garlic and green chillies.
5. Wash coriander leaves in salt water and chop finely.

LET'S START

1. Put mung beans in a pressure cooker. Add salt to it and cook for 4-5 whistles. Keep the flame at moderate level throughout.
2. Separately in a pan, heat 2 tsp olive oil and add cumin seeds to it. As seeds start turning golden, add onions.
3. Keep flame under pan high till the onions turn golden. Add coriander powder and minced ginger-garlic paste. Keep stirring for one minute.
4. Add tomato puree and red chilli powder. Stir and cover the pan. Cook on slow flame for 3-4 minutes.
5. Add this gravy to the mung beans in the pressure cooker. You can add water at this time if the consistency is too thick.
6. Cook in the pressure cooker for two more whistles.
7. Before serving, temper with 1 tsp olive oil and coriander leaves.

GENIUS POWER

INGREDIENTS

For gravy:

1. 300 gm bottle gourd
2. 2 onions, medium
3. 2 tomatoes, red and ripe
4. 1 green chilli
5. 4 cloves garlic
6. ½ tsp turmeric powder
7. 1 tsp extra virgin olive oil
8. Salt to taste

For main:

1. 1 cauliflower, small head
2. 1 yellow bell pepper
3. 2" ginger root, fresh
4. ½ tsp turmeric powder
5. 2 tsp dried fenugreek leaves
6. ¼ tsp black pepper powder
7. 1 tsp extra virgin olive oil
8. Salt to taste

GETTING READY

For gravy:

1. Scrape gently and wash the bottle gourd. Cut into small cubes.
2. Peel and chop onions, garlic and green chilli.
3. Wash and mince tomatoes.

LET'S START

For gravy:

1. Put oil in the pressure cooker and add chopped bottle gourd, onion, garlic, chilli and minced tomatoes.
2. Add salt and turmeric powder.
3. Close the lid and cook on medium heat for two whistles.

GETTING READY

For main:

1. Cut the cauliflower into florets. Scrape and chop stem into small pieces. Soak all in salt water for half an hour.
2. Make a mixture of salt, black pepper and turmeric.
3. Drain the cauliflower and rub this seasoning mixture into the florets.
4. Wash, de-core bell pepper and chop into ½" cubes.

> **NOTE**
> Dried fenugreek leaves are also called 'kasoori methi'. They are used in Indian cuisine and taste similar to a combination of celery and fennel with a slightly bitter bite. Typically, the leaves are crumbled and sprinkled over meat and vegetable curries before serving.
>
> Bottle gourd is a common vegetable also known as trumpet gourd, lauki or doodhi. It has spongy flesh and is a warm season vegetable. This alkaline delight is excellent for the digestive system and is often served when recovering from any fever or infection. Its regular usage removes acidity from the system.
>
> When served in the above combination, it is not visible to children, who usually turn up their nose to this vegetable. It is also a unique blend of summer and winter vegetables. A great balance with nourishing properties.

5. Peel and chop 1" ginger. Cut 1" piece into juliennes for garnishing.
6. Soak kasoori methi in water for 2-3 minutes. Squeeze out water.

LET'S START

For main:
1. Put oil in a pan. Add ginger and sauté on low heat.
2. Add chopped stem of cauliflower and cook for a minute.
3. Add the seasoned florets. Cover the pan and cook on low heat till florets are tender.
4. Add kasoori methi and chopped bell pepper.
5. Mix well and cook for 2 minutes keeping the lid closed.
6. Turn over the kasoori flavoured cauliflower in a dish.
7. From the pressure cooker, take out the bottle gourd and mash well. Pour the gourd gravy over the cauliflower.
8. Garnish with julienned ginger pieces.
9. Serve hot.

TOOTHSOME ROTIS

INGREDIENTS

1. 4 leaves of cabbage, outer dark green ones
2. 4 indian gooseberries
3. 1 tsp bishop's weed seeds
4. ½ cup whole wheat flour
5. 1 cup barley flour
6. Extra virgin olive oil as required
7. Water as required

GETTING READY

1. Wash cabbage leaves thoroughly and keep in salt water for ½ hour. Rinse in running water and chop very finely or coarsely grind them.
2. Wash and de-seed gooseberries. Grate them and mix them with cabbage.
3. Mix both the flours. Add vegetable mixture along with bishop's weed.
4. Knead the dough. Add water only if required.
5. Dough should be of smooth and soft texture.

LET'S START

1. Roll out 4 thin rotis.
2. Use butter paper as a base to avoid them sticking on the surface if required.
3. Cook on medium heat.
4. Remove from the griddle and apply extra virgin olive oil.
5. Serve hot.

GLORIOUS CHICKEN

INGREDIENTS

1. 4 chicken breasts, each skinless and boneless
2. ½ cup bread crumbs
3. ¼ cup hung curd, fat free
4. 1 tsp rosemary leaves, dried
5. 1 tsp basil, dried
6. ½ tsp oregano, dried
7. 1 tsp black pepper corns, powdered
8. 1 tsp parsley leaves flakes
9. Extra virgin olive oil as required

Feast eight: A meal of best ever baked chicken that's succulent to the last bite. Devour with a carrot, sweet corn and raw papaya dish to make it into a filling meal. A salad of choice will go delightfully well to make the meal complete.

GETTING READY

1. Mix bread crumbs, hung curd and seasoning herbs in a shallow bowl.
2. Dip each chicken breast in liquid spread, then in bread crumb mixture.

LET'S START

1. Prepare the baking dish by brushing some extra virgin olive oil on it.
2. Place each breast on the baking sheet.
3. In a preheated oven at 375 degrees, bake the chicken breasts. Turn over after 15 minutes.
4. Bake for approximately another 15-20 minutes or until golden brown.
5. Brush the breasts with a little oil to get that extra brown colour, if required.
6. You have finger licking chicken ready at your place.

SUPERSTAR SWEET CORN

INGREDIENTS

1. 200 gm raw papaya
2. 3 carrots, medium
3. 150 gm sweet corn kernels
4. 2 onions, medium
5. 4 garlic pods
6. 1 tsp sāmbhar powder
7. 1 bay leaf
8. Few sprigs of curry leaves, fresh
9. 1 tsp lemon juice
10. 1 tsp extra virgin olive oil
11. ½ cup water
12. Salt to taste

NOTE
You can vary the quantity of sambhar powder and lemon juice according to your child's taste.

GETTING READY

1. Peel papaya, remove white pith, wash and chop into small cubes.
2. Wash, gently scrape carrots and chop.
3. Peel onions and garlic and cut coarsely.
4. Separately mince onion, garlic and a handful of chopped papaya and carrot cubes.
5. Wash and chop curry leaves and keep aside.

LET'S START

1. Put oil in a pressure cooker. Break the bay leaf into 4 pieces and add to warmed oil.
2. Add minced onion-carrot mixture to the pan.
3. Stir and add water. Cook on low flame for one whistle.
4. Keep cooker in a pan of water to cool it down. Open and add chopped vegetables, salt and sambhar powder. Place back on flame.
5. Cook for 2 minutes on low flame keeping cooker covered with the lid.
6. Add sweet corn and close the cooker to give two whistles.
7. Put off the flame. Allow the cooker to remain closed for a few minutes.
8. Open and remove bay leaves pieces.
9. Stir in lemon juice and dress with chopped curry leaves.
10. Swerve with chicken or fish dishes.

CURRIED BURGERS

INGREDIENTS

1. 2 potatoes, medium
2. ½ cup red lentils, dried
3. 1 onion, medium
4. ½ head cauliflower or 2 carrots, medium
5. 2 cloves garlic
6. 2 tsp curry powder
7. ¼ tsp black pepper, freshly ground
8. Salt to taste
9. ¾ cup whole wheat bread crumbs
10. 4 leaves, green lettuce for garnishing
11. 1 cucumber for garnish
12. 2 tsp extra virgin olive oil
13. 2 tsp purified water
14. Water as required

Feast nine: A twist for the burger loving kids. Fast to make, nourishing, and building the health of your loved ones. The buns are the icing on the top. You can't fail with this feast.

GETTING READY

1. Wash and scrape carrots and dice them. If using cauliflower, break into florets, wash well and soak in salt water for half an hour.
2. Drain florets and chop very finely.
3. Rinse the red lentils and soak them for 4 hours.
4. Wash and boil potatoes whole. Drain water, remove skin and mash well.
5. Peel onion and chop.
6. Mince the garlic.
7. Next, in a saucepan combine 1 cup water and lentils. Bring to a boil. Reduce heat to low.
8. Partially cover and simmer until the lentils are tender, taking care all the water is absorbed. Transfer to a plate; let them cool to room temperature.
9. Wash lettuce leaves.
10. Peel cucumber and cut into slices.
11. Keep both of them aside to be used for garnishing.

LET'S START

1. In a bowl, combine the cooked lentils, mashed potatoes, diced carrots or finely chopped cauliflower.

> **NOTE**
> Avoid using tomatoes with the burgers. The combination of whole wheat buns with raw tomatoes becomes very acidic for young children. Other options for garnish can be sliced onions, gherkins, chopped olives, mint and coriander sauce.

2. Add chopped onion and minced garlic along with curry powder and seasoning. Mix all the ingredients. Use a tablespoon of water if required to get a cohesive texture.
3. With dampened hands, form the mixture into four ½" thick patties.
4. Coat each patty with bread crumbs.
5. Heat oil in a large non-stick skillet over medium heat.
6. Cook 2 patties at a time until evenly browned and heated thoroughly.
7. Serve burgers in whole wheat buns with lettuce and cucumber slices.

SUPER QUICK WHOLE WHEAT HAMBURGER BUNS

INGREDIENTS

1. 3 ½ cups whole wheat flour
2. 1 egg, beaten or 2 tsp non-fat dry milk
3. ¼ cup sugar or 1/4 cup honey
4. 2 tsp yeast
5. 1 tsp salt
6. 1/3 cup extra virgin olive oil
7. 3 tsp lukewarm water
8. 1 cup hot water

GETTING READY

1. Dissolve yeast and lukewarm water in a cup.
2. Combine water, yeast, oil and sugar or honey; let it rest for 15 minutes.

LET'S START

1. Add salt, egg, and flour to the yeast mixture and mix well. Roll out ¾" thick and cut into 10-12 rounds.
2. Place rolls on cookie sheet brushed with extra virgin olive oil.
3. Bake at 375 degrees for 10-15 minutes or until they become slightly brown.
4. Every oven is different. Be careful not to over bake or they will be too dry. When done, brush the top of the rolls with oil.
5. Use these buns to make burgers with other patties like potato pattie, cottage cheese and vegetable pattie as well.

NOTE

These are so quick to throw together. You don't have to wait for the dough to rise twice. Your kids will love the soft texture as they melt in the mouth. Store in plastic bag or a covered container to retain their softness.

7 MIXED BAG

ALMOND MILK

INGREDIENTS

1. 35 almonds
2. 200 ml purified water

GETTING READY

1. Soak almonds overnight.
2. Next morning drain water and peel them.

LET'S START

1. Put skinned almonds in the blender. Gradually add water and churn to make homogenous milk.
2. Blend until the consistency of milk is to your liking. Do not strain the grain.
3. You have now ready a fresh glass of delicious almond milk ready to give your child's body and mind a boost anytime of the day.

NOTE

An excellent source of nutrition and a substitute of dairy milk.

One can easily make almond milk on a daily basis in your kitchen. You can refrigerate it for 2-3 days.

COCONUT MILK

INGREDIENTS

1. 1 coconut, fresh
2. 200 ml purified water

NOTE

You should get about 300 ml milk from a single coconut which includes the nut's water and the purified water added to it. You have the option of adding or decreasing these quantities to obtain your desired consistency. Coconut milk is one of the most nutritious milk on this planet.

GETTING READY

1. Buy a coconut that is large and heavy for its size. This would give you more of flesh and more coconut water which will be sweeter in taste.
2. Break coconut and immediately place it on a sieve to collect its water in a pan below.
3. Keep water aside. Separate the two halves. Remove flesh from the hard woody part of the coconut.
4. Scrape or peel the thin brown skin of the coconut flesh. Wash these coconut pieces under running water.
5. Chop them into small chunks or grate the white pieces.

LET'S START

1. Put the prepared coconut pieces in the blender and churn gradually adding its own water.
2. Add approximately 200 ml purified water to the blender.
3. Now pass this mixture through a white muslin cloth.
4. Squeeze and extract coconut milk.
5. Deep freeze for using this milk anytime you want.
6. You have rejuvenative, natural vegetarian milk ready for use.

TAHINI

INGREDIENTS

1. ½ cup white sesame seeds
2. 2 tsp sesame oil
3. ½ tsp salt

> **NOTE**
> Sesame seeds are an extremely rich source of calcium and are a high protein food. They are a good source of B vitamins and essential fatty acids (EFA).

Tahini paste is made from crushed sesame seeds and has quite a nutty taste. It can be used by itself as a dip with roasted vegetables as well as a spread on bread – a healthy substitute for peanut butter, dairy butter and margarine.

GETTING READY

1. Clean and soak sesame seeds for 4-5 hours.
2. Clean bottle to store.

LET'S START

1. Drain water and rinse seeds once. Place sesame seeds in a grinder and churn.
2. Gradually add sesame oil drop by drop till the mixture is of smooth consistency.
3. Add salt.
4. Pour out in a tightly covered bottle.
5. You can store it for 3-4 days.

COCONUT CHUTNEY I

INGREDIENTS

1. 1 coconut, fresh and medium size
2. 1 beetroot, small
3. 2 indian gooseberries or 2 tsp lemon juice
4. 1 green chilli
5. 1 tsp cumin seeds
6. Black salt to taste

GETTING READY

1. Wash, scrape and chop beetroot. De-seed indian gooseberries.
2. Break coconut and immediately place it on a sieve to collect its water in a pan below.
3. Keep water aside. Separate the two halves. Remove flesh from the hard woody part of the coconut.
4. Scrape or peel the thin brown skin of the coconut flesh. Wash these coconut pieces under running water.
5. Chop them into small chunks or grate the white pieces.

LET'S START

1. Put chopped beetroot and gooseberry chunks in the blender.
2. Add green chilli, cumin seeds and coconut chunks. Blend to a smooth consistency.
3. Add coconut water to attain desired consistency.
4. Add salt to taste and mix.
5. Serve or refrigerate.

NOTE

All sauces and dips can be prepared and kept for 12 hours. For giving optimal nourishment to your child, never use sauces kept overnight

COCONUT CHUTNEY II

INGREDIENTS

1. 1 coconut, fresh and medium size
2. 1 yellow bell pepper, medium
3. 2 tsp lemon juice
4. 1 green chilli
5. 1" ginger root, fresh
6. 2 garlic pods
7. Few sprigs of curry leaves, fresh
8. Black salt to taste

NOTE

All sauces and dips can be prepared and kept for 12 hours. For giving optimal nourishment to your child, never use sauces kept overnight.

GETTING READY

1. Break coconut and immediately place it on a sieve to collect its water in a pan below.
2. Keep water aside. Separate the two halves. Remove flesh from the hard woody part of the coconut.
3. Scrape or peel the thin brown skin of the coconut flesh. Wash these coconut pieces under running water.
4. Chop them into small chunks or grate the white pieces.
5. Wash and chop bell pepper and chilli.
6. Peel ginger and garlic and chop.

LET'S START

1. Put chopped bell pepper and coconut chunks in the blender.
2. Add chopped green chilli, ginger, garlic and lemon juice. Blend to a smooth consistency.
3. Add coconut water, if required, to attain desired consistency.
4. Add salt to taste and mix. Garnish with chopped curry leaves.
5. Serve or refrigerate.

SOYBEAN MILK

INGREDIENTS

1. 500 gm soybeans
2. 1 litre purified water
3. Clean muslin cloth

> **NOTE**
> Soymilk can be kept in airtight bottles in the refrigerator for up to 3 days.

GETTING READY

1. Soak soybeans for 8-10 hours. Drain and add fresh water. Leave it soaked for another 4 hours.
2. Drain and change its water again. Repeat this 7-8 times in total of over 32 hours.

LET'S START

1. Put the beans in a blender and grind to make a fine smooth paste. Transfer bean paste into a clean muslin cloth.
2. Warm one litre purified water in a large pan and dip bundle of soya paste in this water.
3. Raise the bundle out and with a pressing cum rolling motion of the hand, take out milk. Dip again and press. Keep repeating till you feel all milk has been extracted.
4. You will be left with only dry soybean residue with the cloth totally wrung out. Discard residue.
5. You have one litre fresh soymilk ready to be used in delicious recipes.

TOFU - SOY CHEESE

INGREDIENTS

1. ½ kg soybean
2. 1 litre water
3. ½ cup lemon juice

NOTE

You will get approximately 100 gm tofu. To keep tofu fresh for up to 48 hours, place the uncut tofu chunk in a shallow vessel covering it with plain cold water. Tofu has no smell or taste of its own and it adapts to any flavour or herb used in cooking or preparing it. That's what makes tofu so versatile and unique!

Tofu is also available commercially at good grocery stores.

GETTING READY

Prepare soybean milk as given above.

LET'S START

1. Place the milk on medium heat and allow it to come to a boiling point.
2. Now, add the lemon juice. Stir till it curdles. Put off the flame and let it cool for 10 minutes. Strain through a muslin cloth. The solid matter in cloth is fresh tofu.
3. Tighten up the cloth by twisting it. Place it on a flat dish and put a weight on top to make it firm.
4. Remove from the cloth and cut into desired cube size. Refrigerate and use.

8 MAGNIFY YOUR GAINS

FOOD FOR ALL SEASONS – RHYTHM OF NATURE

When your children eat the right foods during each season, you are providing their body with all the necessary nutrients needed for it to face that environment. In other words, seasonal eating puts you in balance. It will not only help restore harmony in their body but will keep them healthy and boost their immune system.

SPRING

After a harsh winter comes spring. When spring comes, it is time to get all those toxins out of the body. Spring is the best time for detoxification. It's the time when your consumption of fruits and vegetables can increase as compared to grains and legumes. High protein foods such as meat and chicken are eaten less often. Spring is a great time to cleanse, revitalize, and rejuvenate your body. Take advantage of it. Prepare yourself for summer.

SUMMER

It's the time for losing lots of water from the body in the form of sweat. Salads and juicy fruits do great during summers. You should replace the fluids lost from the body so it remains hydrated. If you are thinking of getting your kids in shape or getting a makeover done, summer is the best time. Reducing high protein, dense carbohydrate foods and following a pattern of simple foods such as fusion yoghurts, fruit mélanges, sprouts, juices and lots of water will be all that you would need to get them in shape. Summer is activity-time! Go for it!!!

AUTUMN

This season comes with a big change. There is a change in food, in weather, and even in energy. We mostly find harder root vegetables which need cooking. You can have grains, legumes, and high protein meals as a part of your kids food pattern besides the fruits, yoghurt, raitas, and cool drinks. Work their body out until they sweat. Cool down in the pool, or relax with an indoor activity for a change.

WINTER

You need something warm for their body all the time. You can eat cooked foods mixed with salads, sprouts, and balanced with fruits. You can have high protein meals and complex carbohydrates all laid out for your children. Try out vegetables like carrots, potatoes, grains, and squashes. But make sure that they never overeat anything.

Eating in rhythm with the season and hence availability can do more than give your children rejuvenated health.

1. When produce (fruits and vegetables) is in season locally, the relative abundance of the crop usually makes it less expensive. It's the basic law of supply and demand, and when crops are in season, you'll be rewarded financially by purchasing what's growing now.

2. For most of us, the taste of the food we buy is every bit as important as the cost, if not more so. When food is not in season locally, it's either grown in a hot house or shipped in from other parts of the world, and both affect the taste. When transporting crops, they must be harvested early and refrigerated so they don't rot during transportation. They may not ripen as effectively as they would in their natural environment, and as a result they don't taste that good.

3. Foods lose flavour just as they lose moisture when they are held. Fresh, locally harvested foods have their full, whole flavours intact, which they release to us when we eat them. Foods that are chilled and shipped lose flavour at every step of the way – chilling cuts their flavour, transport cuts their flavour, being held in warehouses cuts their flavour. And it's hard to be enthusiastic about eating 5 servings a day of flavourless fruits and vegetables.

4. Foods eaten in season can greatly affect our body's immunity. The resistance to diseases is increased by choosing foods available according to the rhythm of nature.

Determine what's in right now; compare it with the recipes given in the '12 week incredible immunity plan' and dig in. You'll be rewarded with high quality produce, packed with nutrition, at a lower cost. And your children will definitely thank you for it!

WASHING OF FRUITS AND VEGETABLES

Hygiene is prime. All fruits and vegetables should always be washed before consuming them. This is a cardinal rule for your family's health. Besides removing dust and grime, a good wash under running water will effectively reduce the quantity of peel to be removed off the vegetables and make fruits ready for eating.

Most foods are sprayed with chemicals unless you procure organic food. Immerse your green leafy vegetables in strong salt brine for as long as half an hour, then wash under cold running water before using.

Another method to remove parasites and various pesticides from fruits and vegetables is to fill the sink with cold water, and add the juice of 1 lemon and 5-8 tablespoons of salt. Soaking the produce for 10-15 minutes should do the trick. Wash the food well under cold water before use.

Some sprays are poisonous to people who lack the normal digestive acid. For being 100 per cent safe, purchase from your druggist one ounce of chemically pure hydrochloric acid and pour it into three quarts of water. This makes approximately 1 per cent solution and is harmless. Place this solution in a large jar. Simply place the fruits or vegetables in the solution for 10-15 minutes, then remove, and rinse them well with cold water.

ORGANIC FROM INORGANIC

When fruits and vegetables are juiced, most of the chemicals do not adhere to the juice. The chemicals remain attached to the fibre left in the hopper or basket like a magnet to steel. Therefore, it always makes more sense to juice your vegetables. This is the best way to get rid of pesticides and insecticides and get closer to chemical free produce.

Note: All utensils used for serving the food should ideally have a wide mouth especially the glasses. Narrow glasses might look good but due to the size of their mouth, they are not cleaned till the bottom. Over a period of time, debris of food or stagnated water can grow into mould. This will contaminate the food and affect your child's health adversely. If you do use such glasses, always wash with a bottle brush and check before usage.

TOP TIPS FOR CHOOSING FRUITS, VEGETABLES AND OTHER INGREDIENTS

YOGHURT

Mostly, yoghurt is made from either cow, or buffalo, or packed milk. The fat content of all the milks will vary. Packaged milk comes with a specific amount of fat in it and is classified as full cream, toned (skimmed) milk, and double toned (skimmed) milk. Milk obtained directly from the animals requires boiling and skimming manually to reduce the fat quantity.

The taste, texture and flavour of yoghurt made from these milks vary. The tastiest yoghurt is the one made from cow's milk, next is packaged milk, and last is buffalo's milk. Assimilable nutrition content is highest in the same order.

PAPAYA

When buying a papaya, look for smooth skin. If firm, allow to soften at room temperature. It is a delicate fruit and cannot be stored for very long.

GARLIC

Though the garlic bulbs or heads are covered with several layers of a paper-like skin or membrane, the individual cloves are plump, moist, and firm when fresh. Avoid those that appear dried out, blackened, or have green shoots emerging from the tips. These are old and have probably lost their potency. Garlic is best stored at room temperature in a container that allows ample air circulation, such as a basket or a clay garlic pot with holes on the sides. Stored in this manner, garlic will keep well for up to six months. Do not wrap garlic in plastic or store it in the refrigerator where it will mould quickly.

MELONS

Farming of different varieties of melons like – cantaloupe, casaba, honeydew, and muskmelon in different regions has extended its availability all year round. When melons are harvested, they are considered fully matured, or ripe, but still firm. Occasionally, they are harvested too early.

Once they leave the vine, they do not increase in sweetness since they have no starch reserves to convert to sugar. However, they do 'ripen' or soften.

In order to select the perfect melon, learn to recognize the characteristics of ideal ripeness. First, look at the rind. It should have a slightly golden colour rather than a greenish tone. Then, examine the stem end. A slight indentation indicates a 'full slip' or ripeness.

Press gently on the blossom end of the melon. It should be slightly soft. At room temperature, the blossom end should also have a sweet melon fragrance, indicating it is ready to eat. If the melon has a section that is whiter or smoother than the rest of the surface, most likely it's where it rested on the ground during its growing. It shouldn't affect the flavour or quality. Avoid melons with sunken areas that indicate over ripeness and the beginning of mould.

WATERMELONS

When choosing a whole watermelon, look for one that is heavy for its size with a rind that is relatively smooth and that is neither overly shiny nor overly dull. In addition, one side of the melon should have an area that is distinct in colour from the rest of the rind, displaying a yellowish or creamy tone. This is the underbelly, the place that was resting on the ground during ripening, and if the fruit does not have this marking, it may have been harvested prematurely, which will negatively affect its taste, texture, and juiciness.

SESAME

There are distinct advantages to purchasing the 'natural' sesame seeds, those that are un-hulled. The hulls act as a protective coating to prevent rancidity and keep the oil more stable. You can recognize natural sesame seeds by their mottled beige colouring. Because they require no processing, these seeds are priced a bit more reasonably. A good grocery shop or a health food store will most likely have these available.

BROCCOLI

Look for compact crowns that have dark green, blue-green, or the purplish-green, tightly closed buds with dark green leaves that are strong and upright. Intense colours are a good indicator of hearty nutritional content. Yellow or yellowish-green broccoli heads and leaves indicate the vegetable is not fresh and has lost nutrients. Pass on the limp stalks and choose only sturdy, crisp, bright green stems.

Look carefully at the cut ends of the broccoli stalks and choose those that are completely closed. The stalks that have open cores on the bottom tend to be older, woodier, and tougher.

APPLE

Seek out those apples that have not been waxed. Apples keep best and longest when refrigerated. Unrefrigerated apples can become mushy in just two or three days. Purchase them at farmers' markets where you know they have probably been picked the day before market or at supermarkets where they are kept cool. Apples should be firm and blemish-free.

MANGO

They can be purchased when completely hard and stored at room temperature to ripen which can take up to a week. Test them daily with a gentle squeeze. If you plan to use the mangoes right away, apply the gentle squeeze technique to find some that are soft, but solid. If they feel too spongy to touch, they're definitely over-ripe and very possibly spoiled.

When fully ripened, mangoes will give easily to gentle pressure and exude an appealing perfume-like fragrance. You can store ripe mangoes in the refrigerator but not for long. To encourage the ripening, mangoes can be placed in a paper bag at room temperature for a few days. Since this speeds up the process, be sure to test them daily for ripeness.

KIWI

When selecting kiwi fruit, hold them between your thumb and forefinger and gently apply pressure; those that have the sweetest taste will yield gently to pressure. Avoid those that are very soft, shrivelled or have bruised or damp spots. As size is not related to the fruit's quality, choose a kiwifruit based upon your personal preference or recipe need. Kiwi fruits are usually available throughout most of the year.

If kiwi fruits do not yield when you gently apply pressure with your thumb and forefinger, they are not yet ready to be consumed since they will not have reached the peak of their sweetness. Kiwi fruits can be left to ripen for a few days to a week at room temperature, away from exposure to sunlight or heat. Placing the fruits in a paper bag with an apple, banana, or pear will help to speed their ripening process. Ripe kiwi fruits can be stored either at room temperature, or in the refrigerator.

PINEAPPLE

Look for pineapples that are heavy for their size. While larger pineapples will have a greater proportion of edible flesh, there is usually no difference in quality between a small and large sized pineapple. Pineapples should be free of soft spots, bruises, and darkened 'eyes,' all of which may indicate that the pineapple is past its prime. Pineapple stops ripening as soon as it is picked, so choose a pineapple with a fragrant, sweet smell at the stem end. Avoid pineapples that smell musty, sour or fermented.

ORANGE

Oranges do not necessarily have to have a bright orange colour to be good. Whether organic or not, oranges that are partially green or have a brown russet tinge may be just as ripe and tasty as those that are solid orange in colour. Avoid those that have soft spots or traces of mould.

Choose oranges that have smoothly textured skin and are firm and heavy for their size. These will have higher juice content than those that are either spongy or lighter in weight. In general, oranges that are smaller will be juicier than those that are larger in size, as will those that feature thinner skins. Buy organic oranges whenever possible because oranges are among the top 20 foods in which pesticide residues are most frequently found.

DATES

Although dates carry tremendous nutritional values, great care should be taken in their selection because they consist of a sticky surface that attracts various impurities in them. Hence, you should consume only those dates that are packed nicely. Make sure to wash them thoroughly before consuming. This will help to remove the impurities present in them.

CHILIES

Fresh chilli peppers should have a smooth, firm, glossy skin with no soft spots or shrivelling.

CABBAGE

Fresh cabbage has a shiny, crisp look about it. Lift it up to see if it feels solid and compact. Generally, the heavier a cabbage, the denser it is. A standard rule when shopping for cabbage or any vegetable is to avoid those that are wilted, shrivelled, brownish, or looking dried-out. You can be sure that these vegetables have lost their flavour and much of their nutrients from sitting around too long. Resist a tempting sale price if the vegetables don't appear to be fresh.

CARROT

Commercially grown carrots are planted at regular intervals throughout the year, making them available to the consumer all year long. Look for carrots that are bright orange in colour and those that have a smooth skin. Bright colour and smooth texture are indicators of sweet, flavourful carrots. Plump, deep green, attached carrot tops are a true sign of freshness. Carrots with their tops still attached are always sold in bunches. Size does not usually determine the sweetness of a carrot – baby carrots as well as giant ones can be equally sweet. If the greens are wilted and turning yellow or brown, the carrots have lost their freshness and, no doubt, some of their nutrients.

Carrots with a rough, pale, or cracked skin are seldom sweet. A rim of green colour at the top of the carrot indicates it may have become sunburned and will frequently have a bitter flavour. Old carrots can be recognized by their limp, shrivelled appearance. Another sign of an aging carrot is roots that are beginning to sprout along the surface of the skin.

SPINACH

Choose spinach that has vibrant deep green leaves and stems with no signs of yellowing. The leaves should look fresh and tender, and not be wilted or bruised. Avoid those that have a slimy coating, as this is an indication of decay.

Store fresh spinach loosely packed in a plastic bag in the refrigerator 'crisp section' where it will keep fresh for about five days. Do not wash it before storing, as the moisture will cause it to spoil.

CUCUMBER

Choose specimen's with firm, smooth skins, devoid of any blemishes. It's important to look for cucumbers with rich green colour and no soft spots. Cucumbers that bulge in the middle, usually mean are filled with large watery seeds and tasteless flesh. They can be stored in the fridge in a bag for up to ten days.

BELL PEPPER

Choose peppers with firm, shiny, evenly coloured skin. They should feel heavy for their size.

RAISINS

If possible, purchase raisins that are sold in bulk or in transparent containers so that you can judge their quality, checking to see that they are moist and undamaged. When buying raisins in a sealed, opaque container, make sure that the container is tightly sealed and that they are produced, or packaged by a reputed company.

Storing raisins in the refrigerator in an airtight container will extend their freshness and prevent them from becoming dry. Raisins will be most fresh if consumed within six months.

SWEET LIME

The best sweet limes have the skin of an oily, fine texture and are heavy for their size. This type is full of juice with a minimum of seeds and waste fibre. Choose sweet limes of a deep yellow colour for ripeness and sweet taste. They should be firm, but not hard to touch. Avoid the ones that show signs of bruises or any discolouration.

WHOLE GRAIN FLOURS

In order to qualify as a whole grain product, whole wheat or some other whole-grain should be listed as the very first ingredient on the food label. Stone ground is not a requirement for whole grains. If anything, it is a negative as it can introduce sand and other types of stone into your diet.

Even products targeted at the health food market are usually made only with enriched wheat, rather than with whole grain flour. Enriched wheat flour offers no health benefits. Neither does wheat flour. Looks are usually deceiving. Dark brown and black baked goods like breads, muffins, etc. are usually the result of food colouring rather than an indication that they were made with whole grain flour. A vast majority of grain products being sold today are NOT whole grain products.

Choose whole wheat flour, whole barley flour, whole corn flour, old fashioned rolled oats and brown rice, and you will have chosen the best for your children.

BROWN RICE

The difference between brown rice and white rice is not just colour! A whole grain of rice has several layers. Only the outermost layer, the hull, is removed to produce what we call brown rice. This process is least damaging to the nutritional value of rice and avoids the unnecessary loss of nutrients that occurs with further processing. If brown rice is further milled to remove the bran and most of the germ layer, the result is a whiter rice, but also a product that has lost many more nutrients. At this point, however, the rice is still unpolished, and it takes polishing to produce the white rice you are used to seeing. Polishing removes the aleurone layer of the grain – a layer filled with health supportive, essential fats. Because these fats, once exposed to air by the refining process, are highly susceptible to oxidation, this layer is removed to extend the shelf life of the product. The resulting white rice is simply a refined starch that is largely bereft of its original nutrients. Cooking white rice after discarding its soaking water is of little use. The nutrients were already ripped during the refining process.

PRAWNS / SHRIMP

Fresh shrimp should have a firm body that is still attached to its shell. They should be free of black spots on their shell since this indicates that the flesh has begun to break down. If you have the option, purchase displayed shrimp as opposed to those that are prepackaged. The reason for this is, you can smell displayed fish because smell is a good indicator of freshness; good quality shrimp has a slightly salt water smell.

When storing any type of seafood, including shrimp, it is important to keep it cold since seafood is very sensitive to temperature. Therefore, after purchasing shrimp or other seafood, make sure to return it to a refrigerator as soon as possible. Fresh shrimp can last for 1 to 2 days.

You can extend the shelf life of shrimp by freezing it. To do so, wrap it well in plastic and place it in the coldest part of the freezer where it will keep for about one month. To defrost shrimp, place it in a bowl of cold water or in the refrigerator. Do not thaw the shrimp at room temperature, or in a microwave since this can lead to loss of moisture and nutrients.

GLOSSARY

Active immunity – A form of acquired immunity in which the body produces its own antibodies against disease-causing antigens.

Additives – Chemical or food substances added to food products for different purposes: (1) to fortify, or make foods healthier; (2) to preserve, or keep foods from spoiling; (3) to add flavour.

Antibodies – Acting as the body's army, antibodies are proteins generally found in the blood that detect and destroy invaders, like bacteria and viruses.

Antioxidants and Free radicals – Free radicals are 'Wild Bullets' running in your body that cause cell damage. This shooting spree wounds the cells and also converts the affected cell into another free radical. A chain reaction occurs which gets translated into lowered immunity, premature ageing, heart disease, cancer and nervous disorders.

Antioxidants are the compounds that give you protection against this widespread attack. Mother nature has given them as our bulletproof vest. Antioxidants scavenge the free radicals, bind them up, and carry them out of the body. Your most potent supply of antioxidants comes from fruits and vegetables

Aroma – A smell, especially a pleasant, spicy or fragrant one.

Artificial sweeteners – Sweet tasting chemicals that replace sugar in food. Generally, artificial sweeteners add sweetness to food without adding as many calories.

Constipation – Constipation is a decrease in the frequency of stool (the body's waste product) or difficulty in the formation or passage of stool.

Essential fatty acids – EFA's compensate for the assault of free radicals in the cell membrane structure and form a reserve for the cell. Besides playing a central role in cell membranes they also participate in many biochemical processes in the body like the regulation of blood pressure, the elasticity of vessels, immune responses, anti-inflammatory, aggregation of blood platelets, etc. These are commonly classified as omega 3 and omega 6 oils.

Flavonoids – Have been referred to as 'nature's biological response modifiers' because of strong experimental evidence of their inherent ability to modify the body's reaction to allergens, viruses, and carcinogens. They show anti-allergic, anti-inflammatory , anti-microbial and anti-cancer activity. In addition, flavonoids act as powerful antioxidants, protecting against oxidative and free radical damage.

Flavours – Is the sensory impression of a food or other substance, and is determined mainly by the chemical senses of taste and smell.

Fortified products – Foods with nutrients added (synthetic) beyond natural levels.

Immunology – The branch of biomedicine concerned with the structure and function of the immune system, innate and acquired immunity.

Infection – Invasion of the body by pathogenic microorganisms and their multiplication which can lead to tissue damage and disease.

Inflammation – A response of body tissues to injury or irritation; characterized by pain and swelling and redness and heat.

Malnutrition – A condition in which a person becomes sick because he isn't getting enough nutrients. Not only is a malnourished person more susceptible to other diseases, but he may also be extremely underweight and have pale, scaly, swollen, or red skin; bleeding gums; and dull, brittle hair.

Metalloproteins – Metalloprotein is a generic term for a protein that contains a metal ion cofactor. Metalloproteins have many different functions in cells, such as enzymes, transport and storage proteins, and signal transduction proteins.

Microbiology – The branch of biology that deals with microorganisms and their effects on other living organisms.

Epidemiology – It is the study of patterns of health and illness, and associated factors at the population level. It is the cornerstone method of public health research, and helps inform evidence-based medicine for identifying risk factors for disease and determining optimal treatment approaches.

Mucous – Secretion of mucous membranes, normally serving to protect and lubricate many parts of the body. Illness, environmental pollution, smoking, and the consumption of excess fats, sugar, and flour products can stimulate the overproduction of mucous and clog body passage ways, preventing the body from expelling harmful substances.

Orthomolecular science – Coined by Linus Pauling, a double Nobel Laureate, ortho means 'correcting' and molecular is 'at the cell level'. Correcting the chemistry of micronutrients at the cellular level is what this science does. Every food has chemicals in it which go to build the chemistry of the human body. Eating as per orthomolecular nutrition means consuming specific foods in a synergistic way to balance and restore physical harmony. The results are inevitable weight loss, greater energy, strength and youth retention and absence of disease.

Oxidize – Enter into a combination with oxygen. Food elements and nutritive matter gets spoilt when left out in the open after they have been cut. The deterioration in the quantity of nutrients is directly proportionate to the size of the cut food and the time allowed for oxygen to act on it.

Passive immunity – An impermanent form of acquired immunity in which antibodies against a disease are acquired naturally (as through the placenta to an unborn child) or artificially (as by injection of antiserum).

Phytochemicals – Phytochemicals are chemicals found in plants. Plant sterols, flavonoids, and sulphur-containing compounds are three classes of micronutrients found in fruits and vegetables.

Phytoestrogens – A special class of phytonutrients found in plant-based foods. Phytoestrogens have received recognition as a unique health promoting feature offered by whole, natural and nutritious foods. Subsequent experimental research has clearly shown that they are converted in the body to hormone-like compounds that have the ability to modulate estrogen activity.

Supplement – A preparation of minerals or vitamins, usually in tablet form, used to provide additional nutrients to the diet.

Tastes – The sensation that results when taste buds in the tongue and throat convey information about the chemical composition of a food eaten.

Textures – The characteristic of feel or touch. The group of attributes that describes the mouth (oral) feel of a food product. It can be described as thick, gritty, spongy, soft, hard, grainy, dry, creamy, or fatty just to name a few.

Tofu – A white, nearly tasteless blend of soybeans and water from Asia. It usually comes in a dense, congealed square and is smooth and slightly chewy. Not only is it very low in calories, but it is cholesterol-free and high in many nutrients.

Undernourished – Not nourished with sufficient or proper food to maintain or promote health or normal growth. Not given essential elements for proper development even though fed adequate quantities of food.

Vitamin A – An element necessary for growth, healthy eyes, skin, and linings of the throat and digestive tract. Some good sources of vitamin A are eggs, low-fat cheese and dark green, yellow, and orange fruits and vegetables.

Vitamin B1 or Thiamine – An element necessary for the nervous system. Vitamin B1 also helps the body turn food into energy. Some good sources of vitamin B1 are ham, oysters, whole-grain and enriched cereals, pastas and bread, peas, and lima beans.

Vitamin B12 – An element that helps the body use protein, fat, and carbohydrates. It also helps the body produce red blood cells. Some good sources of Vitamin B12 are found only in animal foods such as low fat meat and milk, fish, and oysters.

Vitamin B2 or Riboflavin – An element that helps the body use oxygen. Vitamin B2 is also good for the skin. Some good sources of vitamin B2 are skim milk, low fat meat, wholegrain and enriched breads, dark green vegetables, mushrooms, and dried beans.

Vitamin B6 – An element that helps the body absorb protein. Some good sources are wholegrain (but not enriched) cereals and breads, spinach, green beans, fish, and poultry.

Vitamin C – An element that helps keep gums healthy and hold body cells together. Some good sources of vitamin C are citrus fruits, and dark green vegetables.

Vitamin D – An element that helps the body absorb calcium for strong bones and teeth. Some good sources of vitamin D are low fat milk and other dairy products, salmon, and eggs.

Vitamin E – An element that helps the body produce red blood cells, muscles, and other tissues. Vitamin E also helps protect vitamin A. some good sources of vitamin E are vegetable oil, wholegrain cereals and breads; dried beans, and green, leafy vegetables.

Vitamin – Food element needed by the body for normal growth and function.

Water – The most important nutrient for life, water composes 50 to 60 per cent of our bodies.

Whole grain – A plant food in which the kernel is whole. None of the three parts of the kernel have been removed, like they have in white flour, white rice, and wheat bread. Examples of wholegrain foods are bran cereal, cornbread, oatmeal, whole wheat flour and brown rice.

GLOSSARY FOR COOKING TERMS

Bind – To cause a mixture to hold together.

Blend – To thoroughly mix at least two ingredients together with a spoon, blender or beater.

Brown – To create a brown surface on food with high heat for a short period of time.

Chop coarsely – To cut food into small pieces about 3/16 inches square.

Chop finely – To cut food into very small pieces.

Combine – To mix at least two ingredients together.

Crumble – To break food into smaller pieces with your hands.

Cube – To cut food into small cube shapes, generally about ½ inch.

Dash – The amount of a dry ingredient that is sprinkled in your palm after a few shakes of the container that holds the ingredient, or 1/8 teaspoon or less.

Dice – To cut food into tiny cubes, about ¼ inch.

Dissolve – To mix a liquid and a dry substance until the dry substance dissolves into the liquid.

Dust – To lightly sprinkle with a dry ingredient

Grill – Cook food on a grill.

Grind – To reduce food to particles by using a grinder or food chopper.

Julienne – To cut food into very thin strips or shreds.

Mash – To pound or crush food.

Mince – To cut food into very tiny pieces with a knife or press.

Mix – By using a stirring motion, combine ingredients into a uniform mixture.

Pinch – The amount of a dry ingredient that you can hold between your thumb and forefinger, or 1/16 of a teaspoon.

Puree – To mix food till it becomes a smooth paste.

Roast – To cook by dry heat, usually in an oven, and generally the food is constantly rotated.

Sauté – To cook or brown food quickly in a pan over direct heat usually with a small amount of oil or butter.

Shred – To cut into long narrow strips, generally with a sharp knife or grater.

Simmer – To cook a liquid just below boiling point, bring a liquid to a boil, cover it and turn the heat to low to simmer to create this effect.

Steam – To cook food in boiling water that covers the surface of a pot that is covered.

Stew – To simmer vegetables in their own juices and water.

Stir – To combine ingredients with a spoon in a circular motion.

REFERENCES

Given in this book are many ways that food can behave as common medicine or active compounds to keep you healthy. In all cases the specific pharmacological activity of foods given has been reported by scientific studies. A major source of these studies is the NAPRALERT (NATURAL PRODUCTS ALERT) database which contains more than 100,000 scientific journal articles on the pharmacological activity of plants. Other foods have also been cited because their activity has been included in the large database of medical and scientific publications at the Natural Library of Medicine, or by scientists, and researchers at academic institutions and government bodies.

In some cases the food's active chemicals have been identified as well as the mechanism through which it works. In other cases, even though foods and their constituents exhibit specific health, anti-aging activity, the precise mechanisms is yet to be understood.

BOOKS

The Doctors Book of Herbal Home Remedies – Cure Yourself With Nature's Most Powerful Healing Agents, by the Editors of Prevention Health Books

The Food Bible, by Judith Wills

The Complete Guide to Nutritional Supplements – Everything You Need to Make Informed Choices for Optimum Health, by Brenda D. Adderly, N.H.A.

Healing With Whole Foods – Oriental Traditions and Modern Nutrition, by Paul Pitchford

The Natural Pharmacy – Complete Home Reference to Natural Medicine, by Schuyler W. Lininger, Jr., Alan R. Gaby, MD, Steve Austin, ND, Donald J. Brown, ND, Jonathan V. Wright, MD, Alice Duncan, DC, CCH

The Encyclopedia of Healing Foods, by Michael Murray, ND and Joseph Pizzorno, ND, with Lara Pizzorno, NA, LMT, Prima Publishing, California, 1990

The New Whole Foods Encyclopedia – Comprehensive Resource for Healthy Eating, by Rebecca Wood

Minnie Pandit and Amitabh Pandit, Anti-ageing Exotic Blends, Health & Harmony, 2008

Amitabh Pandit and Minnie Pandit, Superfoods – Make Your Child a Genius, Health & Harmony, 2010

Foods That Heal, H. K. Bakhru, Orient Paperbacks, 1991

Vitamins that Heal, H. K. Bakhru, Orient Paperbacks, 2005

Food Your Miracle Medicine, Jean Carper Simon & Schuster, 1995

Foods That Heal, Bernard Jenson, Health & Harmony, 2001

Natures Known Medicines, Richard Druery and Margie Krick, 1995

Fruit Identifier, Kate Whiteman, Lorenzo Books, 2001

The Complete Illustrated Book of Yoga, Swami Vishnu-devananda, Three Rivers Press, 1988

Heal Again Newsletter, Aparna Levine, Saidas Healing Foundation, 2008

Modeling & Beauty Care Made Simple, Lucie Clayton, Heinemann, London, 1985

Natural Healing From Head to Toe, Aihara, Cornelia and Herman Aihara with Carl Ferre, Garden City Park, NY: Avery Publishing Group, 1994

Sugar Blues, Duffy, William, New York: Warner Books, 1975

Physician Heal Thyself, Faulkner, Hugh, Becket, MA: One Peaceful World Press, 1992.

Let Food Be Thy Medicine, Jack, Alex, Becket, MA: One Peaceful World Press, 1991

How to raise a Healthy Child In Spite of Your Doctor, Mendelsohn, Robert S., MD, New York: Ballantine Books, 1987

The Food Pharmacy, Carper, Jean, Bantam Books, New York, 1988

Food and Healing, Colbin, Annemarie, Ballantine Books, New York, 1986

Tracking Down the Hidden Food Allergy, Crook, William G., Professional Books, Jackson, Tennessee, 1980

Third Opinion, Fink, John M., Avery Publishing Group, Inc, Garden City Park, New York, 1988

Enzyme Nutrition, Howell, Edward, Avery Publishing Group, Inc, Garden City Park, New York, 1985

The Real Vitamin and Mineral Book, Lieberman, Shari, Bruning, Nancy, Avery Publishing Group, Inc, Garden City Park, New York, 1990

Diets Don't Work, Schwartz, Bob, Breakthrough Publishing, Houston, 1982

Hippocrates Live Food Program, Wigmore, Ann, Hippocrates Press, Boston, 1984

The Wheatgrass Book, Wigmore, Ann, Avery Publishing Group, Inc, Garden City Park, New York, 1985

Raw Energy, Kenton, L, Kenton, S., London: Century Publishing, 1984

Nutritional guidelines, Kozora, E.J., Seattle: American Holistic Medical Association, 1987

Fresh Vegetable and Fruit Juices, Walker, N.W., Prescott, AZ: Norwalk Press, 1970

Food, Nutrition and Diet Therapy, Krause, M.V; Mahan ,L.K., Philadelphia: W.B.Saunders, 1984

Nutrition and Diagnosis – Related Care, second edition, Escott-Stump, S., Philadelphia: Lea & Febiger, 1988

The New American diet, Connor, S. Connor. W., New York, Fireside, 1986

Nutritional Influences on Illness, Werbach, M., Tarzana, CA: third Line Press, Inc, 1987

Modern Nutrition in Health and disease, Shils, M. Young, V., Philadelphia: Lea and Febiger, 1988

JOURNALS AND PAPERS

Bianchi, P.G.: Lactose intolerance in adults with chronic unspecified abdominal complaints. Hepatogastroenterology 1983; 30(6):254-57.

Friedman, G.: Diet and the irritable bowel syndrome. Gastroenterology Clinics of North America 1991; 20(2):313-24.

Fritznelis, G.: Role of fructose-sorbitol malabsorption in the irritable bowel syndrome. Gastroenterology 1990; 99:1016-20.

Hunter, J. 0.: Irritable bowel syndrome. Proceedings of the Nutrition Society 1985; 44:141-43.

Hunter, J. 0.: Food allergy – or enterometabolic disorder? Lancet, Augyst 24, 1991: 495-96.

Jones, V. A.: Food intolerance: A major factor in the pathogenesis of irritable bowel syndrome. Lancet, Novenver 20,1982: 1115-17.

Nanda, R.: Food intolerance and the irritable bowel syndrome. Gut 1989; 30: 1 099-11 04.

The effect of virgin coconut oil supplementation for community – acquired pneumonia in children aged 3 to 60 months admitted at the Philippine Children's Medical Center: A single blinded randomized controlled trial, CHEST, October 29, 2008.

Antimicrobial activity of saturated fatty acids and fatty amines against methicillin-resistant Staphylococcus aureus, Biological & Pharmaceutical Bulletin, Volume 27 (2004) , No. 9 1321.

Short term effects of dietary medium chain fatty acids and n-3 long chain polyunsaturated fatty acids on the fat metabolism of healthy volunteers. Lipids Health Dis. 2003 November 17;2(1):10.

A randomized trial of classical and medium chain triglyceride ketogenic diets in the treatment of childhood epilepsy. Epilepsia. 2009 May;50(5):1109-17. Epub 2008 November 19.

Early biochemical and EEG correlates of the ketogenic diet in children with atypical absence epilepsy. Pediatr Neural 1985 March-April;1(2):104-8

Pauline Koh-Banerjeel and Eric B. Rimm: Whole grain consumption and weight gain: A review of the epidemiological evidence, potential mechanisms and opportunities for future research. Proceedings of the Nutrition Society 2003; Volume 62, 25–29.

Jacobs Jr, KA Meyer, LH Kushi and AR Folsom: Whole grain intake may reduce the risk of ischaemic heart disease death in postmenopausal women: The Iowa Women's Health Study. American Journal of Clinical Nutrition 1998; Volume 68, 248-257.

Pamela L. Lutsey, David R. Jacobs Jr, Sujata Kori, Elizabeth Mayer-Davis, Steven Shea, Lyn M. Steffen, Moyses Szklo, and Russell Tracy: Whole grain intake and it's cross-sectional association with obesity, insulin resistance, inflammation, diabetes and subclinical CVD: The MESA Study. British Journal of Nutrition 2007; Volume 98, 397–405.

Frank B. Hu; Walter C. Willett: Optimal Diets for Prevention of Coronary Heart Disease. JAMA 2002; 288 (20), 2569-2578.

Elnima, E.I., et al.: The antimicrobial activity of garlic and onion extracts. Pharmazie 38: 747-748, 1983.

Garbor, M.: Pharmacologic effect of flavonoids on blood vessels. Angiologica, 1972.

Disogra, C,; Groll, L.: Nutrition and Cancer Prevention. Department of Social and Health Services, 1981.

Draper, H.H., et al.: Micronutrients and cancer prevention: Are the RDS's adequate? Free Radical Biology and Medicine 3: 203-207, 1987.

Lo. G.S., et al.: Soy fiber improves lipid and carbohydrate metabolism in primary hyperlipidemic subjects. Atherosclerosis 62: 239-248, 1986.

Robertson, J., et al.: The effect of raw carrot on serum lipids and colon function. Am.J. Clin. Nutr 32(9): 1889-1892, 1979.

Beisel, W. et al.: Single-nutrient effects of immunologic functions. JAMA 245: 53-58, 1981.

Sanchez, A., et al. Role of Sugars in Human neutrophilic Phagocytosis. Am.J. Clin. Nutr. 26: 1180-1184, 1973.

WEBSITES

http://www.otop-nutrition.fr

http://www.csiro.au/org/AnnualReport.html

http://www.doctissimo.fr

Dr. Denice Moffat & Michael Robison, hhttp://www.NaturalHealthTechniques.com

http://www.world'shealthiestfoods.com

http://en.wikipedia.org/wiki/

University of Maryland Medical Center, Center for Integrative Medicine, Alternative / Complementary Medicine Supplements database, http://www.umm.edu/altmed/ConsLookups/Supplements.html